Eli's hand lifted and rested on Aurora's hip, just as her own palm tightened on his arm, almost like she was willing him even closer.

They moved in unison. Lips brushing together for the briefest of seconds before they locked entirely. Her hands wrapped around his neck, the length of her body pressed up against his.

His lips moved across her face to her ear and her neck, and she let out the tiniest groan. He could taste her perfume on his lips, smell it with every inhale.

She let out a breath and stepped back, nervous laughter filling the air between them. Her pupils were dilated, the green of her eyes nearly invisible.

"Whoa," he said, trying to catch his breath.

"Whoa," she repeated, a broad smile across her face.

Dear Reader,

Even though I've been writing for Harlequin Medical Romance since 2011, this is my first vet book! It was so nice to jump into something a little unusual for myself, and I had great fun researching all the different animal conditions you will find in this story.

My grumpy vet is Elijah Ferguson, who is not too happy to take over his father's old practice when there's really no alternative. My vet nurse is Aurora Hendricks and she has an unusual job history that comes back to haunt her. Besides my two main characters, there are some other stars in this book, and for once, they are not children! I hope you love the puppies Bert and Hank just as much as I do, as they help my hero and heroine to their happy-ever-after.

I love hearing from readers, so please feel free to get in touch via my website, www.scarlet-wilson.com.

Best wishes,

Scarlet Wilson

HER SUMMER WITH THE BROODING VET

SCARLET WILSON

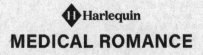

MEDICAL ROMANCE

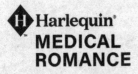

Harlequin®
MEDICAL
ROMANCE

Recycling programs
for this product may
not exist in your area.

ISBN-13: 978-1-335-94247-0

Her Summer with the Brooding Vet

Copyright © 2024 by Scarlet Wilson

Harlequin Enterprises ULC
22 Adelaide St. West, 41st Floor
Toronto, Ontario M5H 4E3, Canada
www.Harlequin.com

Printed in U.S.A.

Scarlet Wilson wrote her first story aged eight and has never stopped. She's worked in the health service for more than thirty years, having trained as a nurse and a health visitor. Scarlet now works in public health and lives on the west coast of Scotland with her fiancé and their two sons. Writing medical romances and contemporary romances is a dream come true for her.

Books by Scarlet Wilson

Harlequin Medical Romance

California Nurses

Nurse with a Billion Dollar Secret

Night Shift in Barcelona

The Night They Never Forgot

Snowed In with the Surgeon
A Daddy for Her Twins
Cinderella's Kiss with the ER Doc

Harlequin Romance

The Christmas Pact

Cinderella's Costa Rican Adventure

The Life-Changing List

Slow Dance with the Italian

Visit the Author Profile page
at Harlequin.com for more titles.

To all the dog lovers in the world. For my own
red Lab, Max, and his partner in crime, our beagle,
Murphy. Best dogs in the world.

PROLOGUE

ELI TRIED TO hold his anger at bay. 'Is that it, then?' he asked his advisers in the room.

His accountant licked his lips, and his solicitor took a breath.

'You have to declare bankruptcy. There's no other option at this point.'

Eli let out the air that had built in his lungs. If it were possible, every cell in his body was exploding right now with pent-up frustration, despair, rage, and part sorrow. All his hard work. All his devotion to opening his own practice and making it a success had now all come to nothing. The countless hours he'd spent doing bone-aching work, concentrating, serving his community, had all been for nothing. All because of a woman.

All because he was a fool.

His solicitor cleared his throat. Eli knew what was coming, and he cringed. 'Your father's practice,' he started slowly. 'The last vet has put in his notice. There are two veterinary nurses. One has worked there for seventeen years. The other has been there eighteen months. The remaining vet is currently undergoing cancer treatment. As of next week, there will be no veterinary cover for the practice, unless you make a new arrangement with other existing practices.'

Eli sighed. He'd never wanted this. Never. His whole life, people had expected him to follow in his father's footsteps and take over once he retired. But that had never been in Eli's plans. No one had been more surprised than he was that he'd actually been bitten by the vet bug. Yes, he'd followed in his father's footsteps and trained as a vet. But from the second he'd started his training he'd made it clear he didn't want to join his father in the family practice.

It had caused many a cross word. But Eli had been determined. He'd served in some larger veterinary practices, gaining experience in small and large animals, taking jobs in the UK, the US, France and Spain. He didn't want to be indebted to his father. He wanted to build his own practice. Eli had always been fiercely independent, even as a child. And now, as a thirty-one-year-old adult, he was back in the situation he'd always sworn wasn't for him.

Would his stubbornness allow his father's practice to fold?

No. It wouldn't.

Being responsible for the demise of two practices would make him unemployable. The vet world wasn't as big as most people thought. Reputation was everything.

'Can you arrange an advert for the practice again?' he asked.

His lawyer nodded, but pulled a face. 'The last advert was out for four weeks. Only newly qualified vets applied. None that have the experience the practice needs.'

'Then maybe I'll need to have a rethink. I could have someone work alongside me for a few months. Get them up to speed. Then, by the time Matt is ready to come back he will be able to take over the supervision.' He pointed to his chest. 'This—me—is only a temporary solution. If we can't find a vet of the calibre we need, then I'll stay as long as it takes to supervise someone new. Get the advert back up.'

His lawyer nodded as Eli stood, staring out across the city. He did *so* not want to do this. But he wasn't too stubborn to see that if he chose to walk away his father's practice would fail, and the people in the surrounding area wouldn't have any care for their animals.

Animals. They always did better for him than people did.

And that was the simple reason he would do this—for the animals.

CHAPTER ONE

Aurora Hendricks tugged at the edge of her uniform as she juggled the puppy in one hand and her keys in the other. The little guy had wriggled so much her uniform had started to creep upwards, revealing a sliver of skin at her waist. Not exactly how she wanted to meet any potential new clients.

She gave the puppy a rub at the top of his head. 'Hold on, little guy. We'll get you in here and I'll check if you've got a chip. I'm sure someone is missing you very much.'

As she'd driven to work this morning, the car in front of her had swerved and screeched its horn. Aurora had caught sight of the terrified puppy darting across the road and had immediately pulled over.

Ten minutes of tramping through muddy woods, leaving a trail of treats and keeping very quiet, had allowed her to coax the very frightened little guy into her arms.

He didn't look quite so frightened now, and

the mud on his paws, and her shoes, were leaving both a trail on her uniform and on the floor.

'Are you always late? And in such a state?' came the sharp voice to her side.

She turned her head sharply. Standing inside one of the rooms was a tall, lean-looking man, with light brown tousled hair, longer on top, that unshaven but trendy look, and an angry expression on his face.

'And who might you be?' she asked, equally sharply. All her senses had gone on alert. She was supposed to be opening up this morning. There shouldn't be anyone else here—and certainly not someone who was a complete stranger.

'I was about to ask you the same thing,' he responded.

She blinked and took a breath, trying to still her racing heart and stave off her fight or flight response. In her head, she was calculating how quickly she could put the puppy somewhere safely and find something to whack this guy around the head with. There was a broom in the corner. That would do.

'Since I'm the one with the keys,' she said sharply, 'and the uniform—' she looked down at her smudged pale pink tunic '—I guess I'm the one to ask questions. Since when did you think it was a good idea to break into my practice?'

She said the words, but she didn't get the vibe

from the guy. He didn't look like some random thief. In fact, the more she looked at him, the more she was inclined to stare.

He was kind of handsome. In an annoying kind of way.

The one thing she definitely wasn't getting was a fear factor—which she could only presume was good. Because—due to past experience—Aurora Hendricks had developed a spider-sense when it came to danger, and men.

She placed the bedraggled puppy on the table near her and kept one hand on him as she shrugged off her wet jacket.

'So, this is *your* practice, is it?' Her head shot back up as she contemplated letting the puppy go for a second to grab the microchip scanner in the nearby drawer. There was an amused tone in his words. It raised her hackles and irritated her.

She held the puppy with one hand and put a few treats in front of him as her other hand grabbed the scanner. 'Well, until someone else shows up it is,' she muttered. Then paused. 'What? You're not some other random locum, are you?'

A furrow creased his brow. 'What do you mean—another random locum?'

She ignored him, concentrating on scanning the puppy. She checked all the usual spots where microchips with the owner's details were usually inserted on puppies, with no success.

'Oh, dear,' she sighed, picking up the puppy and holding him close to her chest as she stroked him. 'You must be an escapee.'

The man moved forward. It was as if she'd captured his attention. 'An escapee from where?'

She gave a sorry shrug. 'One of the puppy farms. There's a few about here. If he's not chipped, they hadn't managed to sell him yet.' She held the puppy up and squinted at him. 'Or maybe he's not from the puppy farm. He doesn't look like a pure breed.'

The man gave a nod as he looked appraisingly at the puppy. 'Maybe some kind of collie cross?'

She blinked. 'You *are* a new locum, aren't you?' Then she wrinkled her nose. 'But how did you get a set of keys?'

'They're mine.'

Her nose remained wrinkled. He reached over and took the puppy from her hands. 'Let me check him over.'

She'd been too slow to keep a hold of the puppy, but her instincts around animals were strong. She put her hand over his. 'No, you don't. Not till I see some proof of who you are, and your credentials.'

He looked at her in surprise. 'So, you're not bothered about being in here with a perfect stranger, but I tell you I'm checking a stray and you want to see my credentials?'

She couldn't tell if he was angry, annoyed or a mixture of both. But she didn't care.

She looked him up and down. 'I think I could take you,' she said frankly. 'I've learned how to take care of myself over the years. But I'll fight you to the death before I let you near that puppy without checking out who you are.'

They stood in silence for a few seconds, looking at each other, like some kind of stand-off.

Then he gave a nod and gestured for her to follow him. He walked slowly out to the hall and stopped in front of a picture on the wall.

She turned to face it, even though she'd seen it and walked past it a million times. It was of the original owner, David Ferguson, with his fellow vet partner, and his son.

The man raised his eyebrows at her.

And the penny dropped.

She squinted at the picture and moved right up close to it. 'That's you?' she asked incredulously.

She didn't mean it quite the way that it came out. But the skinny-looking kid in a T-shirt and ill-fitting jeans was a million miles away from this over six-foot lean guy with light tousled hair, pretty sexy stubble and blue eyes. She looked even closer at the picture, and then back to his face again.

'You might have the same hairline,' she said finally.

He made a noise that sounded like an indignant guffaw. 'Elijah Ferguson,' he said. 'Son of the late David. I'm only here until Matt is well enough to come back to work, and we can recruit a new vet to take over.'

Aurora was still thinking things through. 'Matt mentioned that you were a vet.'

She'd actually felt instantly relieved when he'd said the name Matt. Because that meant that he knew who usually worked here. This wasn't just some elaborate ploy to break into a vet's and steal some drugs, or an abandoned puppy.

'Where are you staying?' she asked.

'In the adjoining house,' he said quickly. 'But I plan on including that in the advert for the new recruit.' He nodded upstairs. 'I can sleep in one of the rooms upstairs while I train him.'

'Or her,' she said automatically.

'Or her,' he agreed with a smile, before holding up the puppy and looking him in the eye. 'Now, do I have your permission to check this little guy over?'

'I suppose,' she said, unsurprised when he walked straight through to one of the consulting rooms behind him. It was clear he knew the layout of this place. He'd obviously spent a large part of his life here.

She accepted that he was who he claimed to be. But it still didn't explain him just turning up like this. She was an employee. Didn't she have a right to know what was going on? It seemed rude.

She watched him cautiously. Aurora might not have been a vet nurse for too long—only four years so far. But she was wise enough to know if someone was competent or not.

He sounded the puppy's chest. Checked its mouth, eyes and ears. He had a little feel of the tummy and ribs, standing the puppy upright to check its gait. Then he got out the scales and weighed the little guy.

Her hands were itching to take the puppy from him. She wanted to check it over herself. It wasn't that she didn't trust him to do his job, it was just that she didn't *know* him.

Why didn't he work here? Wouldn't it have made more sense to work alongside his father, then take over from him? Maybe he wasn't that good a vet—and his father, from what she'd heard, had exacting standards, hadn't wanted to work alongside him.

Or maybe this guy was one of those fly-by-night vets who locumed everywhere before it was discovered they just weren't that good.

All of this flew through her head as she

watched him examine the puppy, as she filled the deep sink with warm water.

'He's scrawny,' came the deep voice.

'Well, that's obvious.' She could tell that from first sight, and from forty metres away.

'Heart murmur,' he added, and her heart gave a little pang.

'Severe?' Her skin had already prickled.

His eyes were still on the puppy. He shook his head. 'No. I'd want to recheck on a regular basis, but I suspect it might just disappear as he grows.'

She walked over and held out her arms. 'My turn. Let me clean him up, and then give him some food.'

'What've we got?'

She lifted the puppy, who didn't object as she gently submerged him in the few inches of warm water, lifting a soft cloth to remove the dirt and stones from his coat and paws. She named the two brands of food they currently had in the cupboard, and Grumpy vet scowled. 'Is there a deal with them?'

She was trying not to smile. 'Grumpy' vet had just automatically come into her head, rather than his actual name. She let out a sigh. 'I don't know. It's been stocked here since I arrived last year. We sell some over the counter.'

He picked up his keys, and it struck her that she hadn't seen a car out front. 'I don't like it.

I'm going into the city to pick up some other supplies. I won't be long. Don't feed him until I'm back.'

Aurora gave a nod. Dog food could be an endless debate. Some practices had deals with brands to stock their food, and usually received some sort of incentive to do so. She hadn't been involved in any of this. There were websites and chat forums that dedicated hours to the nutritious content of every food on the market and the benefits of raw, dry or wet dog food. What she did know was the practice also had a freezer stocked with chicken and plain white fish—which they frequently used for sick dogs, alongside some rice, or sweet potato. If Mr Grumpy didn't get back in time, she would happily make something up for the little guy.

A few moments later she heard a car engine, and looked out to see a low bright red sports car emerge from the garage next to the house. The same car was in one of the other photographs on the wall. It must have belonged to Elijah's dad.

She finished cleaning off the puppy, before giving him a few more treats and settling him in a basket with a blanket in one of the secure stations in the main observation room. He was already half asleep; clearly his escapee adventure had been too much for him.

Aurora went upstairs and changed into a spare

uniform, before coming back down, turning the sign on the door to open and checking the answering machine.

There were a few routine appointments this morning. Weight checks, nail clipping, eye drops and a skin treatment for a West Highland terrier. She also had a few test results to check from samples that Matt had taken last week before he'd had to stop working. Elijah Ferguson hadn't told her what exactly he was doing here, so she didn't want to make any assumptions.

As the first patient came in, she settled into her normal routine. Finding this practice on the outskirts of Edinburgh had been a blessing in disguise. At twenty-eight, vet nursing hadn't been Aurora's first job. She'd had stars in her eyes as a kid and gone to stage school, getting a few small TV roles, then a lead as a daughter in a new series about a family that had gone to Africa. Funnily enough, the main character in the series had been a vet, and her whole time in Africa had been spent among staff who had great respect for animals.

The series had catapulted her into stardom and onto social media, with pictures of her in clubs with friends, or shopping in London, regularly appearing in the tabloids. Soon after that, the stalking had started. It had taken her a little while to realise at first that the letters delivered to her agent, then the gifts that had mysteriously appeared at her rental, were actually a bit more sinister. As they'd moved into the second TV series, where staff changes made her uncomfortable, and had led to a member of the crew sexually assaulting her, Aurora had quickly realised she wasn't going to continue. Her colleagues had been supportive and leapt to her defence, particularly when the press called the incident a publicity stunt around #MeToo. Her return to London had coincided with the arrest of her stalker after an apparent kidnapping attempt and Aurora was all out of showbusiness.

Her saving grace had been the friends she'd made first time around in Africa, and one of the show's vet advisors had encouraged her to look at vet nurse courses. It had been exactly what she needed. Her course in Hertfordshire, along with some hair dye and returning to her own name, had given her the time and space she'd needed to escape the demons that had chased her. A few of her colleagues had eventually recognised her along the way, but she'd always managed to shy away from talking about her experience, or why she'd left.

Her first year after her degree had been spent at a practice on the edges of London. But when she'd seen this job advertised on the outskirts of Edinburgh, and realised the practice worked with both domestic and farm animals, it had seemed a perfect match for her.

Her old-style cottage was tiny, but she'd bought it outright with her earnings from the TV series. The bills were reasonable, and she was able to keep saving. Life, for the most part, was good now, as long as she could continue to keep out of the spotlight.

She finished checking the weight of a cat whose owner had been told to put the cat on a diet for strict health reasons. It seemed it was an uphill battle. 'Ms Bancroft?' Aurora asked. 'Have you been sticking to the food we talked about?'

The older woman nodded solemnly while not quite meeting Aurora's eyes.

'And no treats?'

The woman's face screwed up and she gave a minimal shrug of her shoulders. 'She only gets a few.'

The cat glared at Aurora—actually glared at her, as if she knew exactly what they were talking about and didn't approve in the least.

'Well, Trudie's weight is still the same. She really needs to lose some. Her bones and joints are under so much strain while she's this heavy, and her heart too.'

The elderly woman lifted her indignant cat back into her arms. 'Well, I'll try my best.'

Aurora gave an inward sigh. 'The good news is that she's not put any more weight on. So, that's at least a step in the right direction. How about you bring her back in two weeks and we'll check her again?'

Aurora could almost sense that Trudie had Ms Bancroft exactly where she wanted her, and likely annoyed her most of the day for treats.

'Two weeks.' Ms Bancroft nodded, before allowing Aurora to put Trudie back into her cat carrier as she hissed in annoyance.

Next, Aurora trimmed a Pekingese's nails, clipped a hamster's teeth, gave eye drops to a young kitten with a nasty infection, and finally treated a white Highland terrier with atopic dermatitis. She gave careful instructions to the young owner. 'Around twenty-five per cent of West Highland terriers develop atopic dermatitis at some point in their life. We need to keep on top of it, as it can cause skin damage, infection and general discomfort. It's really hard to get them to stop scratching. If you treat the skin like this every day, it should reduce the itch, and help keep the symptoms at bay.'

The young girl nodded seriously. Aurora knew that she loved her dog, and would do her best to treat the condition.

By the time she'd finished with the fourth patient, Elijah Ferguson still hadn't returned. She quickly made some chicken and white rice for the puppy, cutting the chicken into tiny pieces before taking him outside to let him relieve himself. 'We need to give you a name,' she said, taking a snap on her phone and uploading it to the vet website page, asking if anyone knew the owner.

She held the puppy up. He'd cleaned up well, his black and white coat almost fluffy at this stage. She studied him for a few seconds. 'Bert,' she said with a smile. Her favourite cast member back on the show. Old enough to be her grandfather, and the person who'd stepped in when needed. It had made a big difference for her, and she'd always be grateful. 'You look like a Bert,' she said to the little guy before sitting him back on her lap whilst she checked some of the test results from samples taken last week. The first result made her close her eyes for a second and take a few breaths.

Cancer. In an older dog. And fairly advanced. The dog had recently developed a limp and the owner had brought him in to be checked. Matt, the vet she'd been working with, had been fairly sure what the diagnosis might be, and had already prepared the owner.

But Matt wasn't here. His own treatment for cancer had taken its toll, and he'd needed some rest and recuperation. Frankie, the French vet who'd worked here up until last week, had put in his notice and gone to work in Dubai.

Aurora knew the owner of this dog. He'd lost his wife a few years ago, and she wanted to make sure she dealt with this sensitively. From first meet, she wasn't entirely sure that Elijah Ferguson was the person to do that.

She picked up the phone, and kept a hold of Bert, as she made the call. It was the one part of her job that she didn't enjoy, but she knew it was one of the most important. So she ignored her heart thumping in her chest and took a deep breath as the phone was answered.

Eli was mad. And there was no real reason for it. He was mad about puppy farms around the vet practice. He was mad about the fact his own car had broken down last night and he'd been forced to use one of his father's. Just driving it now brought back a whole host of memories. He was mad about not contacting the practice staff before he'd arrived. A novice mistake. He'd startled that woman this morning and it was hardly a good start.

He was even mad about the brand of food that Matt had obviously chosen to sell these last few years—even though it was entirely none of his business.

He could actually feel the suspension on the

low-slung sports car suffering due to the amount
of different feed he'd just purchased from a sup-
plier.

And he was mad about how remarkably attractive the vet nurse was. Her dark red hair had
been windswept and strewn about her face, her
uniform dirty, and his first reaction wasn't entirely gracious as she'd walked in with the dirty
puppy. But it seemed that she was unfazed by
his bad temper.

It suddenly struck him that he hadn't even
asked her what her name was and he groaned
at his pure bad manners. That sent off another
wave of annoyance in his head at how disappointed in him his father would have been.

Truth be told, the second that Elijah Ferguson had even glimpsed the familiar countryside
every part of him had been on edge.

There wasn't even a reasonable explanation
for it. And he knew it. It wasn't as if he'd had
an unhappy childhood or been abused in any
way. His mother and father had both loved him.
But his father had been obsessed with his job.
He'd always been working long hours, tending
to horses or sheep on farms at three in the morning, missing Eli's football matches because of an
unexpected emergency. Falling asleep at school
assemblies because he'd been up all night. Everyone had loved David Ferguson, including Eli.

It was just hard to tell anyone how it felt to literally have an absent father. Always feeling second best to a job. Joining his dad as a young kid at the practice on a Saturday had been the only way to get a part of his attention.

Even as an adult he hadn't really been able to articulate it. So it just hung above his head, as words always unspoken, feelings never really being acknowledged, and a part of himself feeling resentful and stupid. He'd had a good life. His father had been delighted by his career choice. He'd been so proud of Elijah being top of his class.

And all of that had just made Eli want to run further and further away.

Today, as soon as he'd set foot in the place, he'd been jittery in a way it was impossible to describe. Again, he felt foolish. His father had been dead for six years now. But memories of him were all over the place. The photos. The colour of the walls. The layout of the practice. Matt hadn't changed a single part of it.

As he turned back towards the large country practice, he finally paid attention to the little blue car parked in front. It was covered in mud. Clearly the nurse had gone off the road to recover the puppy. He remembered the fierce look in her eyes as she'd demanded to know his credentials, as she'd clutched the puppy to her chest.

He liked that. He admired that. And the thoughts caused a gut punch to his stomach. Last time he'd had his attention drawn by a member of staff he'd practically sold his business down the river. That was the last thing he'd ever do again. The last.

He pulled up alongside the car and walked back up the stairs to the entrance. It was later than he'd planned and as he opened the door he could hear her talking on the phone in a low, sympathetic voice. 'I'm so sorry,' she was saying.

He frowned. What was going on?

Something made his footsteps slow, and he heard other parts of the conversation. Test results. A cancer diagnosis. A poor prognosis. Alarm bells started going off in his head.

Who on earth was this woman, and what on earth was she doing?

'Who are you talking to?' he demanded as he walked inside the room.

She started, and the puppy, which was on her lap, gave a little jump.

'Just one of our clients,' she said. 'They were waiting for some results from tests that Matt took last week.'

Her green eyes were wide and he'd clearly surprised her.

'And you think it's your job to do that?'

He could see her bristle. She turned her head

away from him and continued her conversation on the phone. 'Mr Sannox, our new vet has just arrived. I know this is really upsetting for you. Why don't I drop by later and I can tell you everything you need to know?'

'You won't,' snapped Eli. It was all he could do not to pull the phone from her hand. She was really overstepping. And what was more, he hadn't even asked her name so he could actually demand that she stop right now.

'Finish that call.' His hands were on his hips right now. This shouldn't be happening. Not in his practice. News like this should always be delivered by a vet. She had absolutely no right.

But whatever her name was, she completely ignored him, actually standing up and putting her back to him as she continued to talk. 'Yes, I'll see you about three o'clock. No problem at all.'

If he hadn't noticed the tiniest tremble of her hand he would be yelling right now.

She put down the phone and turned to face him, eyes blazing. 'I was right about you.'

It was the last thing he'd expected her to say. 'What?'

'I actually contemplated if I could rely on you to give results like those. And guess what? I thought not. And I was entirely right. How dare you interrupt me when I'm telling someone their pet is going to die? What's wrong with you?'

She was angry now. Her jaw was clenched.

'What's wrong with me? What's wrong with you? What gives you the right to think you should be giving results like that without them being checked by a vet first? Do you even understand the results? Do you know the treatment options? Are you qualified for any of this?'

Oh, no. A horrible thought crept over him. This woman had demanded to know his credentials earlier—he hadn't even thought to ask about hers.

Not only did he not know her name, he didn't know if she was qualified in anything.

His brain was going mad. The logical part screamed, *The lawyers told you the two vet nurses were qualified.* One of them he'd known for ever. This one...? Had she been here a year? Two? He couldn't remember.

She stepped right up under his chin. 'Let's get things straight right now, Elijah Ferguson,' she said, an unexpected accent appearing in her tone. 'You don't ever talk to me like that again.' The words were hissed. 'You left here, after appearing this morning, not even telling me where you were going, when you'd be back, or even if you were going to be working here in future. As far as I know, *I'm* the only qualified person on shift today.' She pressed her hand against her chest. 'I know these people. I know exactly how much Rudy means to Mr Sannox, and I know exactly what's happened in his life these past few years. I have a duty of care to him, and to his pet.' She flung her hand to the ceiling. 'So, you go off and worry about pet food, while I deal with the patients and tell them the news they don't want to hear.'

Her accent, which had started as a mere hint, was now pure Liverpudlian. The anger which had also started as a hint was now emanating from every pore of her body.

'Jack Sannox?' he said, his skin growing cold.

She blinked in surprise and nodded. 'Yes.'

Lead was settling in his stomach. 'I know him,' he said automatically. 'This is his dog?'

'His border collie.' Her words were careful. 'He lost his wife a few years ago. He's become quite solitary. Something happening to Rudy will kill him.' The words were dramatic. But it seemed that Aurora had learned rapidly about farmers, their livestock and their pets.

'So, you've told him,' Eli repeated.

She looked at him carefully with those calculating green eyes. 'I've told him,' she said, holding his gaze. 'Because from what little I saw of you this morning, didn't give me confidence you would treat the case with the compassion it deserves.'

Wow. She wasn't messing about. Could he really work with this woman—even if it was for only a few weeks? He was instantly annoyed and offended. But should he be?

He straightened his own back and shoulders and held out his hand towards her. 'Elijah Ferguson,' he said. 'But call me Eli. Qualified eight years ago. I might not appear a very good human, but I can assure you that I'm an excellent vet.' He let out a long stream of air from his lips. 'And I know Jack Sannox. I went to his wife Bessie's funeral.'

His hand was still hovering in midair. She hadn't moved yet.

She'd changed since he was out, and her tunic was now a pale green, complementing her eyes. Her previously scruffy hair had also been combed and pulled back into a neat bun at the nape of her neck. She looked much more professional, and what was more, she had an extremely professional air. It was something that most people couldn't quite put their finger on. But she had it.

And though he was reluctant to say it, the fierce protection he'd now witnessed for both animals and owners was actually what he looked for in a colleague.

She still hadn't shaken his hand. There was tension in the air. They certainly hadn't started on the right foot. He wasn't even sure if this situation could be retrieved.

He brazened it out. 'I'll be working here for the near future. In the meantime, we're trying to recruit a new vet. If I have to take someone newly qualified I will, then hopefully mentor them for a short while to get them up to speed until Matt is well enough to come back and work alongside them. So, in effect, for a short period I'll be your new boss.'

Her shoulders tensed at those last words. He could see a million things flash in her eyes. And he was pretty sure one of them was her resignation. Considering this practice was currently losing staff like a dandelion shedding seeds in the wind, it wasn't what he wanted to hear.

Finally, she stepped forward and shook his hand with a firm grip. 'Aurora Hendricks,' she said, her accent vanishing once more. 'I've been here eighteen months, and it's always been a team approach. I'm not much for hierarchy. And yes, I am fully qualified. I have a BSc in Veterinary Nursing, and I know exactly what those test results mean.'

Aurora. An unusual name. But it suited her. There was something else though. Something strangely familiar about her that he couldn't quite place. Had they met somewhere before?

A little quiver of something ran through him. With her dark red hair, pale skin and green eyes, she was certainly attractive. He was sure if he'd met her before she would have made an impression. So, what was it about her that was familiar?

She took a deep breath, letting the words she'd said settle before she continued. 'And I don't just mean the science of the results. What I mean is, I'll likely be going up to Jack Sannox's farm for the next year to keep an eye on him.'

And that was when he knew.

That was when he knew that he had to find a way to work with this woman.

He needed her beside him, not against him.

He nodded. 'Aurora. It's an unusual name.'

She looked surprised that this was where the conversation was going. 'Well, "call me Eli",' she said, as quick as a flash, 'Elijah isn't so normal either.' She glanced out of the window. 'My father named me. After the actual Aurora Borealis. Aurora means dawn.'

He gave her a rueful smile. 'Well, my dad named me too. And he wasn't religious, but he remembered the name Elijah from Sunday School as a kid, and just liked it. I'm probably lucky he didn't name me after his favourite breed of cow.'

'Angus or Galloway?' she quipped.

He rolled his eyes. 'More than likely something neither of us have ever heard of.' He took a careful breath. 'If you don't mind, I'd like to familiarise myself with Rudy's case, then I'd like to go with you later today to speak to Jack. He will need extra support, because it's likely there will be no treatment that will actually make a difference.'

He turned his attention to the puppy in her arms. The little guy hadn't even squirmed during their exchange, just watched everything with his big brown eyes. He leaned forward and smiled. 'What are we going to do with this guy?'

'This is Bert,' she said determinedly.

'Where did that name come from?'

She shrugged. 'A reliable friend. I've posted a pic on our website. But since he's not tagged, I'm assuming he isn't actually owned by anyone. We might need to see if the local shelter can arrange someone to foster or adopt.'

'What about any of our clients?'

'What do you mean?'

'Is there anyone that might be looking for another dog? A companion for another dog?'

Aurora looked thoughtful and then wrinkled her nose. 'We've had a few older clients die in the last few months, and myself and Anne have managed to place their pets with other clients.'

She sighed. 'I think we might have used up our supply of local, willing pet fosterers.'

He reached over and took Bert in his arms. 'He looks about eight weeks. Puppies take a lot of work. Maybe he already had an owner who just wasn't ready for the work involved.'

It only took a few moments to make a decision. 'Let's give it a few days on the website and see what happens. I'll vaccinate him, and in the meantime he can stay here with me. There were kennels outside at one point, I'll go and have a look and see what state they're in.'

'You're staying here?' She seemed surprised.

He shrugged. 'I told you earlier, I could move into the house but it doesn't seem worthwhile. I want to use it as an incentive for the new vet. I'll just sleep upstairs. There's three bedrooms, a living room and a bathroom. There's even been a new kitchen put in.'

'You do know that if we take a patient overnight, either myself or Anne usually stay in one of the other rooms?'

He tucked Bert under his arm. 'You do?'

She nodded.

'It's okay.' He shrugged. 'I'm sure we can make it work. It'll only be for a few months. And I don't snore,' he added.

She arched her eyebrow. 'But I do.'

And there it was. Another challenge. It seemed

that Aurora Hendricks was someone who was going to keep him on his toes.

He leaned down and nuzzled into Bert. 'Let's go find some earplugs, kid. We've got to plan ahead.'

CHAPTER TWO

THE RAIN WAS pelting down as Aurora arrived the next morning, and the normally paved area in front of the practice was swimming in mud. She turned and frowned at the nearby hillside. There had been some slippage in the past—was it going to happen again?

She shucked off her wellies at the front door, knowing she had some flat shoes in her locker—and promptly stepped in a pool of puppy pee.

'Ew,' she said before smiling. It wasn't the first time, and wouldn't be the last.

'Sorry,' came a voice from the doorway. Eli had Bert tucked under his arm. 'We tried the kennels last night after I'd fixed them up but—' he looked down at Bert '—it seems that Bert is actually a house dog.'

Aurora couldn't help but smile. She peeled off her wet socks and walked across the tiled floor, rubbing Bert's head. 'Are you just showing him who's boss?' Bert licked her hand. 'Guess you'd

better get started with the toilet training then,'
she said.

He looked down at her painted toenails. 'How
about I get you a pair of socks first?'

She nodded gratefully, and was pulling the
thick woollen socks onto her feet as Anne came
through the door.

'Typical Scottish summer,' said Anne, shaking
off her umbrella, and then stopping short. 'Eli?'
she said in wonder, before crossing the room in
long strides and enveloping him in a giant hug.

Aurora's gaze flicked from one to the other.
Anne only worked here three days a week now.
But she'd been here from the time that Eli's dad
had run the practice, so it was obvious that they
would know each other.

Eli, surprisingly, returned the hug with a relieved expression on his face. Had he been worried that Anne wouldn't be happy to see him?

'Who is this?' she asked, rubbing Bert's head.

'A stray, we think,' he said, glancing over at
Aurora. 'This is Bert. I'll keep him for the next
few days to see if anyone comes forward.'

'Sure you will,' said Anne, still smiling. She'd
released him now but tucked her hand into his
arm. 'Let's just go and have a cup of tea and
catch up a bit. You can manage, can't you, Aurora?'

Aurora gave a nod. Eli looked a cross between

still being relieved along with a mad dash of panic. 'Can you put Jack Sannox in the diary for later today, since he wasn't up to it yesterday?'

Aurora gave a nod as Anne swiftly moved Eli through to the kitchen, talking the whole time.

She checked through the patients for the day. She noticed that Eli had put a few notes next to some, mainly questions on getting some more information from owners or looking at medications or treatment plans. She took her time to read them all. He was thorough. He'd also left some notes and instructions about the surgical list for tomorrow, asking her to call all the owners to remind them of the instructions for their pets, prior to any procedure.

Aurora always did that automatically, but he wasn't to know that so she tried not to let it annoy her and just left it for now.

She sighed as she looked at a few of the notes he'd left regarding Rudy and Mr Sannox. Jack had called back and asked them to change their visit until today. He'd said something about needing a little time.

In all honesty, she would have preferred to see Jack yesterday, if anything, just so she could give him a hug. Aurora finished what she was doing and tried not to be curious about the conversation that was clearly going on in the kitchen.

She'd have loved a cup of tea but didn't want to intrude.

She'd always enjoyed working with Anne, who came equipped with a million stories and a world of expertise. She lived in the nearby village and had never even considered working somewhere else. Aurora could remember a few times when Anne had casually mentioned that it was a shame that Elijah hadn't taken over from his father, but had always backed the words with something like 'children should always spread their wings'.

An unexpected arrival—a cat with fleas, brought by a horrified owner who asked a myriad questions about her designer wardrobe and furniture—kept her attention away from the conversation in the kitchen. Aurora spent a considerable amount of time concentrating on treating the cat and emphasising how important it was to continue treatment, before covering the basics about vacuuming the home, washing all bedding and soft furnishings and spraying everything with flea spray.

After that, there were some routine appointments. Anne and Aurora shared the vet nurse appointments, accompanying Eli when required and keeping an eye on Bert.

Anne opened the store cupboard and blinked at the newly stocked food. She leaned over and checked the side label before giving an approving nod. 'This one is hypoallergenic. It will actually suit a lot of our patients with more sensitive tummies.'

Aurora smiled. She hadn't even looked that closely. 'So, what do you think of our new vet?' she asked, trying to sound innocent.

She could tell that Anne was bursting to talk. Anne had lots of skills but keeping secrets wasn't her best—although she could, when necessary, be discreet.

'I'm so happy to see Eli again,' she said with a smile. 'He's grown up to be the picture of his father.'

'Has he?' Aurora had seen the photo on the wall earlier, but didn't think they were so alike.

'Oh, yes,' said Anne with authority. 'Same height and build. Eli has his mother's colouring, but his mannerisms are identical to his father's.' She gave a soft smile. 'It brings back lots of memories.'

Aurora wondered how many questions she would get away with. 'His father and Matt were partners, weren't they?'

Anne nodded. 'Right up until David retired. He worked on much longer than he should have. But by then Sarah, his wife, was dead and Eli was away working someplace else. He didn't want to leave Matt on his own.'

Aurora looked out over the Scottish country-side. Right now, it was difficult to get a good view, with the sheeting rain and small mudslide from the hills nearby. But usually this view was a wild array of green, a dash of some heather and a few spots of white sheep.

'Why on earth is it so hard to recruit around here?'

Anne gave a sorrowful shrug. 'I'm not sure. I think for a while David was too picky, and Eli seems to have inherited his father's traits. When the practice passed to him, he constantly didn't think any of the applicants were good enough.' She gave Aurora a knowing glance. 'You know the thing—he didn't want to work here, but no one else was good enough?'

Aurora frowned as she tried to make some sense of her new workmate. 'Interesting.' She paused, looking in the direction of the kitchen to make sure the coast was clear, and then asked the ultimate question. 'So, why did Eli never come back to work with his dad, or take over?'

Anne wrinkled her nose. 'He'd opened his own practice for a while on the outskirts of London. Not sure what happened there. I guess right now it's just about timing. Matt's sick and Frankie's left. What other option did he have?'

And that answer left Aurora with an uncom-fortable feeling. Anne was going to retire soon.

But Aurora had another twenty years or more to work. If they couldn't recruit another vet, this practice might fold. She didn't want to end up out of work. She loved her cottage and where she lived. She didn't want to have to move. But if Eli was only there on a temporary basis, she might need to consider other options.

Anne nodded towards the car park as another car pulled in. 'Recognise them?' she asked.

Aurora shook her head, 'No idea.'

Eli met her at the front door. As soon as he stood next to her, she got a waft of his aftershave. Fresh but woody, it made her breathe in even deeper. Darn it. The last thing she needed was to be attracted to someone she worked with. Particularly when he could be occasionally snarky. Mixing work and pleasure was never a good idea. It didn't help that he glanced sideways at her and gave her a half smile.

A couple in their twenties entered the practice with a cat carrier. Although they didn't have an appointment, there was a short gap where they could be seen. Eli showed them through to one of the examination rooms. Aurora instantly had a weird feeling. She watched the interaction between the couple as they removed their cat from the carrier and placed him on the examination table.

Eli asked them some details as he examined

the cat, which was called Arthur. Again, as she watched him, she appreciated how thorough he was. But something about the couple seemed off. It was that niggling feeling right between her shoulder blades that she really couldn't explain to anyone. Aurora had had this before—it sometimes caught her by surprise.

The man seemed to continually talk over his partner. He also kept glancing towards Aurora, even though she was not speaking to him directly. She was merely making notes on the computer as Eli examined the patient. His continued glances made her nervous and uncomfortable; he even hinted at a smile a few times towards her when he knew his partner was looking elsewhere. There was just something creepy about him.

She could sense that Eli caught something in the air. He gave her a curious look but continued with his examination, and after a few careful questions Aurora knew exactly where this diagnosis was going. Eli looked at them. 'I think I can say with some confidence that Arthur has diabetes. All the symptoms you've described—the weight loss, the excessive drinking and excessive eating—all point in that direction. I only need to run a few minor tests to be able to confirm it.'

The women looked pale. 'Is this serious?' she asked.

Eli nodded. 'It can be. But diabetes in cats is not uncommon and it's a condition we can treat.'

'Will he need injections?' asked the guy. 'My gran has diabetes and she requires injections.'

Eli nodded again. 'That's very likely. Why don't you leave Arthur with us for a few hours, and when you come back we can confirm the diagnosis and make a treatment plan?'

The guy shot another few glances in Aurora's direction and she shifted uncomfortably in her seat. She hadn't spoken a word to him during the consultation, so knew that she had done nothing to attract his attention.

'Is everything all right?' asked Eli as soon as they left.

Aurora gave her shoulders a little shake. 'Just something about that guy. He made me uncomfortable.'

She didn't want to go into any details. Being assaulted, and then being stalked, had a huge influence on her life. The outcome of these had affected both how she lived her life and her decision-making. It had been built into her TV contract that she would be covered for any consequences from being in the TV series. She knew that essentially had been around any possible accidents or injuries but, thankfully, her assault had also been covered—and not for a short period of time. Now, all these years later, she still attended counselling sessions when she needed them. They'd started intensely but now happened as and when Aurora ever decided she needed them. She had that odd prickly feeling that she'd be making contact with her counsellor some time soon.

She stood up and walked over and picked up Arthur. 'How about I get started on those tests for Arthur and you can prescribe his insulin?'

Eli gave a nod and started taking more notes. Aurora half hoped that only the woman would come back. She would need to spend some time with Arthur's owners to explain his new diet plan, and how to do his injections. They'd already left insurance details, so she knew Arthur would be covered, and it would likely take another few visits to get his condition stabilised.

It had been a strange start to the day. Eli had been nervous about seeing Anne again and wondered how she might act. But Anne had been warm, friendly and professional. He just had a sense, deep down, of a slight feeling of disappointment that emanated from her. It could all be in his head—maybe it was just old feelings being rehashed?

Anne had been well aware of the underlying

hostility that lay between Eli and his father. But she showed no hard feelings towards Eli, and seemed happy to see him.

He still wasn't entirely sure about Aurora. She'd seemed a little off in the earlier consultation, but maybe he was just misinterpreting things.

He was still trying to get to grips with how the practice was run. It seemed that Anne and Aurora shared the variety of roles, and he wondered if that was the best use of their time. Aurora had mentioned the practice being a team approach. It was hard to get a sense of that when he was the only vet. And he wasn't sure how much time and energy to invest in finding out, when he would only be here a short space of time.

But Aurora intrigued him. He could sense something from her earlier when she'd been uncomfortable in the consulting room. He'd almost felt a shift in the air. He was slightly annoyed that he hadn't picked up on anything, but would pay better attention in the future. He still wanted to find out a little bit more about her and her experience. His eyes were continually drawn to her, no matter how hard he tried for them not to be. His brain was constantly wondering about her. And it was odd, but he could sometimes swear there was a buzz in the air between them. But maybe he was just imagining it.

He wondered if he would get that opportunity to find out a bit more about her when they visited Jack in a few hours' time. But in the meantime, he had other things to concentrate on.

Bert was showing no interest in toilet training. It had been so long since Eli had looked after a puppy that he'd forgotten how hard it was. He cleaned up a variety of puddles and took Bert back outside with some treats to try and encourage him to toilet outside and reward that behaviour. No matter where Bert eventually ended up, he would likely need to be toilet trained, so it was worth the extra time and effort. More people were likely to adopt a puppy if they knew the toilet training routine had started.

Anne shouted them all through to the kitchen, where they all prepared lunch. She looked at the visits for the day. 'What is going on at the Fletchers' farm?' she asked.

Eli looked up. 'What do you mean?'

Anne put her hand to her chin and looked thoughtful. 'It's in the book for today but there's no notes next to it. I'm sure that Matt has already been there a few times. I think some of the cattle have been poorly—but I don't think there was anything specific.'

'I have no problem going back up there,' said Eli. 'Has Don Fletcher phoned down again?'

Anne shook her head. 'The writing in the

book is definitely Matt's. He must've put a note on here a few weeks ago that he wanted to go back.'

Eli was thoughtful for a minute. 'Put it forward a few days, please. I want us to spend a bit of time with Jack Sannox this afternoon.'

Anne nodded and changed the diary. Lunch was quick, and Eli spent a bit of time checking off everything he would need for the few surgical procedures that were scheduled for the next day. One lesion to be biopsied. One cat, and one dog to be neutered.

Aurora's answers were swift to each query. 'Done, done, and done.'

He got the hint that she was getting annoyed with him. But this was basic stuff. He didn't know Aurora, and had no idea what her capabilities were. Last thing he wanted was for an animal to present tomorrow who hadn't been properly prepared for surgery. Then it would require cancellation and would be a waste of time for all concerned. He was only ensuring every box was ticked. It was what any good vet would do. If Aurora didn't like it? Too bad.

The afternoon passed quickly and soon it was time to do the home visits. For farms, it went without saying that the vet had to visit. For domestic animals, home visits were much fewer. Occasionally when an animal had reached the end of their life span, and was clearly in pain or desperately unwell, some owners would ask for them to be put to sleep at home, rather than in the practice. Eli knew that Matt and his father always respected the client's wishes in these cases, and he would do the same. He pointed at a name on the list that had been scored out. 'What's happening with this one?'

Aurora took a deep breath. 'Mrs Adams wants another day. She says she's not quite ready.'

He took a quick glance at the notes. An elderly cat, signs of dementia, untreatable cancer, now being incontinent, and its back legs weren't functioning. 'Are you sure she can cope?' When an animal reached this stage it was like being a full-time carer. It could take a lot out of owners.

Aurora pressed her lips together and gave a tight nod. 'She'll cope. She'll phone us back when she's sure she's ready.'

'Does she have pain relief for her cat?'

'Of course, we would never leave any animal in pain.' There was a tiny bit of defensiveness to her words.

'Okay then, ready?' he asked as they made their way outside to head to Jack Sannox's farm.

'We can't go in that.' She smiled, pointing at the low-slung sports car. 'Have you seen the farm roads?'

He pointed to the garage. 'Don't you know

my dad was a bit of a car fiend? He's got another three in there. There's an old eighties Land Rover. It's built like a tank and it's fit for any farm road. He used it for most of his visits while he worked here.'

The car wasn't modern enough to have a key fob press-button lock, so Eli had to do the old-fashioned way of opening the doors with the key.

Aurora climbed in. Part of him wanted to get to know her a little better. He couldn't deny how attractive she was. And she didn't wear a ring. But that meant nothing these days. After his previous experience, the last thing Eli wanted to do was have any kind of relationship with a member of staff. So why was he even having these thoughts? He couldn't deny how attractive she was, but she was prickly at times.

As the thought entered his head, he almost laughed out loud. Prickly? So was he. More than prickly. But he couldn't help it. Being back at the family home and practice was conjuring up a whole host of past feelings—ones that he really hadn't wanted to deal with. And now? When, if he didn't recruit another vet, the whole place would be under threat didn't seem like the best time to deal with things.

As she sat in the Land Rover next to him, the scent of her perfume drifted towards him. Hints of amber and musk. Quite distinctive. Her hair, which had been tied up earlier, was now down around her shoulders. The long, dark red bob suited her, and looked more sculpted that he would have expected.

'What?' she asked unexpectedly.

His stare had clearly been noticed. He decided to play things out. 'How long have you been here?'

'Eighteen months,' she answered easily.

'And what brought you to Scotland? Was it family? Or did you get married?'

She gave him a distinct side-eye. 'I'm not married. No partner. This practice brought me to Scotland.'

So, the fact he'd been asking if she had a partner had not been lost on her, and he pretended not to be secretly relieved.

'You came here for the job?'

'Of course I did.'

'Where did you train?'

'Hawkshead.' The Royal Veterinary College. The most prestigious place to carry out vet training, or vet nurse training.

'Outside of Edinburgh is a long way to travel.'

She shrugged. 'I don't have family ties, and I'd worked already in outer London, I wanted to move to a place where there was a chance to work with both domestic and farm animals.'

He gave a smile as they continued along the

winding country road. 'Not a lot of people want to work with both types of animal.'

She waved a hand at the clothes she'd changed into. Big green wellies and a large, dark waterproof coat. 'I don't like to be caught unawares. We're going to talk to Jack about Rudy, but if there's another farm issue he wants us to look at, I like to be prepared.'

Eli couldn't help but be a little impressed. He'd stashed his own stuff earlier in the back of the Land Rover. It was nice to know that Aurora was prepared too.

'What about your accent?' he asked. 'I've noticed it tends to come and go.'

For a moment there was silence, and he wondered if he'd stepped over a line he shouldn't have.

'My accent?'

He swallowed. He'd started the conversation. He couldn't back out now. And, for some reason, he wanted to know. His head flooded with thoughts about his past experience. Could Aurora be pretending to be someone she wasn't? Was there a reason she changed her accent at times? He needed to be able to trust those he worked with.

But as she brushed a length of her hair behind her ear, and he caught a glimpse of her pale skin, his stomach clenched. She was anxious. Anxious he found out something she was trying to hide?

'Yes,' he said firmly. 'Most of the time you don't seem to have an accent at all. But occasionally the odd twang seems to slip in.'

'The odd twang?' she repeated. This time he could see her eyebrows raised. She looked as if she were about to roast him.

'Yip,' he said with a smile in his voice as he turned onto the road towards Jack's farm.

'My accent does come and go,' she said carefully. 'I grew up in Liverpool. But when I worked in London some of the clients appeared to have an issue with my accent, so I tried to tone it down.'

It was an odd kind of explanation. London was one of the most diverse populations in the UK, with a multitude of accents. But he did concede that certain parts of London had old-fashioned clients who might be a bit haughty towards a Liverpudlian accent.

'No excuse for behaviour like that,' he said promptly. 'I've worked all over the world. I get that my Scottish accent can be quite broad, and I've had to repeat myself on numerous occasions, but I wouldn't try and hide my accent.' He shot her a glance. 'If I'm in another country, I usually get mistaken for Irish instead of Scottish. But I can live with that.'

They pulled up outside Jack Sannox's cottage. The word cottage was a bit of a stretch. The farmhouse was much more impressive as it had been extended over the years, but the original parts of the cottage were still there. He obviously took pride in his home.

Eli took a breath. 'Wow… Haven't seen this place in years. He's extended—it looks great.'

Aurora climbed out of the Land Rover. 'I've only been here once before, when there was an issue with the pigs. Matt said the work had just finished and Jack gave us a full tour. He was very proud.'

'So he should be.'

They moved to the front door and Jack opened it with a solemn expression on his face. He led them through to his sitting room, where Rudy was lying on a rug on the sofa. Jack sat down next to him.

'How's he been?' asked Eli, bending down so his face was next to Rudy's and stroking his head.

'He was up last night whimpering. I don't think the painkillers are working.'

'I can increase them,' said Eli instantly. 'But it may make Rudy drowsy.'

'He's so used to being by my side, walking the fields with me, riding the tractor,' said Jack, a definite waver in his voice. 'He's just not going to be able to do that.'

'No, he's not,' said Eli reluctantly. He wanted to give Jack a realistic expectation for what happened next.

Jack sighed and stared out of the window, one hand on Rudy.

Aurora moved and sat beside him, taking his other hand in hers. 'It's not fair. And we know that. None of us deserve the dogs that we have—they're all just too good. I know this time of year is difficult. I know it's around the same time that your wife died.'

Jack's eyes widened in surprise; he turned to look at her. 'But you never got to meet Bessie.'

'I know, and I'm sorry about that. But you're the one I need to worry about.'

Jack blinked and Eli could see the wetness in his eyes. 'No one left to worry about me,' he whispered, and Aurora leaned over and gave him a hug.

'That's not true.' She looked over at Eli. 'I'm sure we can make Rudy comfortable, and give him another few months.'

Part of Eli wanted to be annoyed. But the way she was looking at him with those green eyes was almost sending him a secret message. He had written in Rudy's notes that he thought he could make the dog comfortable for the next few months. Maybe she was just letting him know that she was following his lead?

Jack turned to him. 'I don't want my dog in pain. Are you sure there isn't anything else that can be done?'

Eli spoke in a low, serious tone. 'His cancer has spread. Some of the organs that are affected could give him other symptoms. But most of these we can control. I can certainly control his pain. There's another medication we can try—a cancer medication that can also shrink some of his tumours and give him a better quality of life.'

Jack gave a sniff. 'A few months, you say?'

Eli nodded. 'I'll talk you through the medications. I brought them with me.' He moved back over and kneeled in front of Rudy again. 'I think you'll do okay as a house dog, Rudy.'

Rudy looked at him with his big brown eyes, and Eli remembered why he was a vet. For this. To take care of animals that had brought joy to families and give them a comfortable end to their life.

He looked at Aurora, who still had one hand in Jack's, her other arm around his shoulder. She was squeezing it. It struck Eli that he didn't know who might have hugged Jack since his wife had died a few years ago. This could be his first hug since then.

He also wasn't sure how Aurora had found

out about when his wife had died. Maybe Matt had told her? But however, she'd found out, she'd taken the information into consideration when here. He liked the fact that she'd thought about the whole situation, and not just the immediate circumstances.

They left Jack nearly an hour later. They were quiet. It was always sad when discussing plans for a terminal pet.

Aurora leaned her head against the window. 'I'm not sure if Rudy will want to be a house dog.'

'I'm not sure either,' admitted Eli. 'But we'll just have to play it by ear, and give Jack the support he needs.'

She turned her head towards him and locked her eyes on his. 'This,' she said quietly. 'This is part of the reason I wanted to move. You get to know these patients. You get to know what matters to them. In the city, it was just a constant stream of French bulldogs, dachshunds, cockapoos, cavapoos and chihuahuas. Most of the time we never saw them on a regular basis. We didn't get to form any kind of relationship with people. The turnover was incredible.'

'And you decided that wasn't for you?'

She gave a nod. 'Or maybe I just like cows,' she said with a smile.

There was something in that smile. Something

that made him know that she was being entirely honest.

But as soon as he had that thought, something else flashed into his head. But was he really a good judge of character? After all, he'd thought his last practice manager, Iona, was honest. He'd been sucked in by everything she'd said. They'd even started dating. Then the bills had started to arrive. It seemed that money from the practice had been funnelled off into places it shouldn't go—mainly Iona's bank account.

She'd offered to take over the wages system, the banking, the accounts. In other practices, it was a fundamental part of the practice manager's role. She'd come with excellent references—which he'd later found out had been faked—and he'd been thankful for the assistance.

It wasn't until another vet in the practice had taken him aside about an unpaid bill, that he'd found one day when he came in early, that Eli had any understanding at all that something was amiss.

And as the world had come crashing down around him, and his staff had been forced to find other jobs, and Iona had disappeared just as quickly as she'd appeared, Eli Ferguson had been left feeling like a complete and utter fool.

It seemed that fraud was harder to prove than he'd first thought, particularly when it seemed that it was his signature on some of the accounts. He'd had to dig into what little of his savings he still had to engage experts to confirm that he hadn't signed for certain things. Loans and credit cards had been the most popular. But that was the reason for his earlier visit to his accountant and solicitor. He'd had no option but to file for bankruptcy.

He wouldn't be able to be a real financial partner in his father's practice for a number of years. Instead, he would have to be an employee. And if he was embarrassed about that it was just too bad.

So maybe his judgement couldn't be relied upon at all. Not when it came to business or financial matters.

And any thoughts of how attractive Aurora Hendricks was, how cute her smile, the shine of her hair, or the fact she was feisty, with a warm heart, he had to put clean out of his head.

He was only here on a temporary basis. And he would do well to remember that.

CHAPTER THREE

AURORA STILL HADN'T quite got a handle on her new boss. She didn't want to admit she found him a little intriguing. He was handsome, there was no denying it, with his tall frame, his tousled light brown hair and his blue eyes. That darn designer stubble made her palms itch to touch it. If she'd met him at a bar somewhere she would definitely be interested. But their initial meeting had been a bit unusual.

In a way, she was glad that he'd caught the sharp side of her tongue and how protective she was of her work space, and any animal in it. That was important to her.

Then there was the fact she'd been uncomfortable around that cat owner the other day. He didn't need to know why. But her spider-sense never tingled without good reason. She'd learned to trust her instincts. It had been part of the reason she hadn't really panicked at their own first meeting. Eli might be a bit untouchable, but he wasn't intimidating or threatening.

She was still unsure about her job security though. Whilst vets might be hard to recruit in this part of the country, it seemed that the population around Edinburgh had veterinary nurse as a first career choice. Jobs were usually sought after. She'd been lucky when she'd interviewed for here. Both Anne and Matt had been in the middle of an emergency surgery—a dog who had developed a blockage in their bowel. It was a surgery she'd been involved in before and she'd offered to roll up her sleeves and assist so to speak. They'd hired her shortly afterwards and she'd been happy here.

The outskirts of Edinburgh was also a good place to hide. But hiding? Was that what she was actually doing?

Half of her hoped that no one remembered her fifteen minutes of fame. But, like any TV series, the show had ended up streaming on some of the satellite services and gained new fans. Every now and then she saw a social media post about *Where are they now?*

No one had ever got her location right. But there had been a few sightings—particularly when she'd qualified as a veterinary nurse and started working just outside London.

She wanted a private life. She didn't want to be dragged back into the #MeToo debate. She'd stood up for herself at the time, and now wanted to just get on with the rest of her life. She no longer had an agent. She'd drifted away from the fellow cast members on the series, and most of the crew. She'd changed her mobile number, and since her Equity card was under her acting pseudonym she'd felt relatively safe.

Of course, there was the inevitable person she'd gone to school with who occasionally commented on her disappearance from the TV screens, but most people thought she'd headed to find fame and fortune in the States, and failed. She was actually happy for that rumour to continue. It meant that life was safe, in this little part of the world.

The world didn't really understand the damage she'd suffered. The assault had left her feeling vulnerable and frail. The stalking had left her feeling unsafe. She'd had to build herself back up, take advice, attend regular counselling. Self-defence classes with regular refreshers helped too. But, most of all, she trusted her instincts. She would make sure she was never alone with that new client on any occasion. It didn't matter what reason she gave to Anne or Eli—she might even just tell them the truth. She'd learned to believe in herself, and that was what she'd do.

Today was going to be a bit different. She'd told Eli that she was interested in working with farm animals, and today they were doing several visits to farms.

'Are you really ready for this?' asked Eli as he climbed into the old Land Rover.

'Are you?' she asked, glancing at their list. She wrinkled her nose. 'Have you met all these farm owners before?'

He shook his head. 'I only know one out of three. I've been on two of the farms before, but one of them has changed hands.'

She gave him an amused glance. 'I've checked the notes. We have mysterious cows at the Fletchers' farm, temperamental pigs at the Sawyers' and a possible lame horse at Jen Cooper's riding school.' She gave an approving nod. 'It's going to be a good day.'

He gave her an amused sideways glance. Maybe he hadn't quite believed she did love farm work. Well, he would soon find out.

They ended up going to the Sawyers' farm first as it was closest. Shaun Sawyer took them to his pigsty, where two of the pigs had been separated out from the others.

It was clear that neither of these pigs were happy. They were grinding their teeth, were listless, with lots of abdominal kicking.

'Any vomiting?' asked Eli, as he prepared to go into the sty.

Shaun shook his head. 'Only minimal. And not for the last few hours.'

Aurora prepared herself too, and Eli gave her a sideways glance. 'I don't suppose they've escaped at all?' she asked as she swung her leg over the fence. The field around the pigsty had some straw but also a decent amount of mud. Aurora wasn't bothered at all.

Shaun pulled a face. 'They did a few days ago. Five of them did. But we managed to get them back relatively quickly.'

She jumped down, just as Eli did, and moved over to the nearest pig. She followed his lead and they both checked for any obvious bloating or signs of intestinal blockage. 'This one is a bit tachycardic,' she said.

'Mine too,' said Eli. They both checked the pigs' temperature, and Eli walked back over to Shaun. 'My gut feeling is this is colic. You've got an automatic feeder in action to stop gorging, plenty of water and plenty of space for the pigs to move around. There's no sign of obstruction at present—but you know that can be rapid. It could be they've eaten something that doesn't agree with them when they escaped. There is always a higher risk of twisted gut as we come into the summer and temperature fluctuates. But I don't think that applies right now. If we think there's an obstruction we might need to X-ray or ultrasound them.'

Shaun frowned and shook his head. 'Can I watch them a bit longer?'

Eli nodded. 'You can call me if you have any concerns. I'll give you some non-steroidal anti-inflammatories for them both.'

'Where did they go when they escaped?' asked Aurora.

Shaun inclined his head. 'Over the field and into the school playground.'

'Ah,' she said with a smile. 'Any chance they raided the school bins and overdosed on some sweet treats?'

Shaun pulled a face. 'My pigs? More than likely.'

They stayed a bit longer, observing the pigs for any signs of something more serious, before finally getting ready to leave. As Aurora went to swing her leg over the fence, there was a loud squelch and her foot came over, leaving her welly boot stuck fast.

The momentum carried her, and she landed on the other side of the fence with a laugh.

Eli shot a careful glance at Shaun and then they both burst into laughter too. Eli was still in the pen, so made his way over to her boot. He had to grab with both hands to finally free it, and nearly landed in the mud himself.

By the time they'd rinsed their wellies and got back into the car they were still laughing.

'What's next?' asked Aurora.

'You choose,' he said. 'Horse or cows?'

'Cows are my favourite farm animal,' declared Aurora. 'So let's leave them to last and go and see the horse first.'

The journey was only fifteen minutes and as the countryside sped past Aurora settled a little more comfortably into her seat.

'Where did you work before?' she asked.

As soon as the words were out of her mouth she realised it might not have been a good idea. He bristled. He actually bristled. Then he took a breath and said quickly, 'I've worked all over. I worked in Madrid for a while, then in Brittany in France, three months in Italy, then in the US in Florida and Maine, and in Lincolnshire in the UK.'

'Wow!' said Aurora, feeling part admiration and part envy. 'That's a huge range of countries.'

'I went for the experience with the animals.' He gave a smile and raised one eyebrow, as if he was just admitting something. 'In Madrid I worked in a practice that specialised in horses. Brittany was mainly farms. Florida—'

'Tell me it was alligators!' she interrupted.

He laughed. 'I did encounter one on a golf course, but not through work.'

'Darn it,' she muttered, then frowned. 'So, what was it in Florida then?'

He gave her a sideways glance. 'Turtle rehab.'

Her eyes widened. 'You're joking, aren't you?'

He shook his head. 'Are you telling me you don't think turtles should have care too?'

She stuttered for a moment. 'Oh…of course I don't think that. It's just such a change.'

'Working with sea life was such a great opportunity. I jumped at the chance. When I moved to Maine it was a real mix again. I was part of a practice with forty vets. I saw domestic animals and dairy and beef cattle, equine and poultry.'

Aurora couldn't take her eyes off him. 'It's like you stuck one finger in an atlas to decide which country to go to, and one finger in Pasquini to decide what animals to look after.'

He waggled a finger. 'Not all animals are in Pasquini.'

'True,' she admitted. Then she gave him a sideways glance. He seemed much more relaxed around her now. Less defensive. She wondered why he'd bristled at first. 'That must have been a lot of exams.' She knew that vets had to sit country specific exams to get the licence to practice.

He groaned. 'You have no idea. Thankfully, exams have never really bothered me.'

'Just as well,' she said as they turned into the riding school and pulled up outside the stables.

Jen Cooper stuck her head from one of the stalls and walked quickly over to meet them, getting straight to business. 'Thanks for coming. It's Bess. I noticed this morning her gait was different. It's her right leg. She was fine yesterday, and there's been no accident.'

'No problem,' said Eli as he held out his hand. 'Eli Ferguson. I've got a bit of experience with horses, so let me have a look.'

'Where did you get your experience?' said Jen casually as she opened the stall door.

'Jerez,' he said simply.

Aurora stopped walking—as did Jen. 'Jerez?' they both said in unison.

The school was renowned for the world-famous Andalusian horses that danced in shows.

Both heads turned towards him, and Eli held up one hand. 'What I'll say is that those horses are kept in pristine conditions, have the best veterinary care and some of the best facilities I've ever had the pleasure to work in.'

Aurora hid her smile. She knew exactly why he might think they would comment. Some people didn't like animals used in a show, or sport for that matter, and queried the conditions and attention.

Somehow, she knew every word he said was true. She might have only known him a few days but she already had a real sense of the man and his values.

'What about the bulls?' asked Jen, her gaze narrowing.

Eli shook his head. 'I had no involvement with any of the bulls in the vicinity. My sole area was the horses. The equestrian school was very clear to make sure all who dealt with them knew they had no part in any of the bullfights or any of the bull runs that happen.'

Jen gave him a careful look. 'Okay, let's go and have a look at Bess then.'

Eli worked steadily, using the scale that some veterinary surgeons used to grade lameness in horses. He wasn't afraid to get up close and personal and once he was sure that Bess was steady and not upset he waved them over as he examined one of her hooves, picking it out with a hoof pick, checking for foreign objects, sharp stones or nails. 'Tell me a bit more about this morning,' he said to Jen.

'No problem. Out in the paddock as normal. Then out for a gallop late morning. She was fine until lunchtime yesterday.'

'Hard ground or soft ground?' His head was still dipped over Bess's hoof, his blue eyes peering carefully at her as he gently examined her.

'There's a very slight purplish-red spot,' he

said. 'I think this might be a stone bruise. Do you have any pads you can use while this heals?'

Jen gave a swift nod and headed towards a large box in the stables. 'It goes without saying Bess will need to rest, and I'm happy to come back and take another look in a few days.'

Aurora looked over at Jen, who she hadn't met before. 'Do you know what to look for? Inflammation, formation of a haematoma or an abscess?'

Jen gave her a serious nod. 'I'll get our farrier to come over and balance the hoof and remove the shoe for now.'

They talked for a few minutes more as Aurora stood on the sidelines. It was interesting to watch how Eli worked. It was true, he did have a good deal of knowledge about horses, and for a few moments she wondered if Jen and he were testing each other.

But then she quickly realised he was just trying to get a feel for how experienced Jen was, and what kind of treatments he could recommend to her, knowing she could carry them out safely.

The batting back and forward between the two was interesting, and Aurora started to have a good sense about his experience. At first, it had seemed all flash, sitting so many exams, working in so many countries, with such a range of animals; he'd seemed a bit like a child in a sweetie shop who couldn't decide which to try first.

But now she wondered if it was just a genuine thirst for knowledge. And what made it even more irritating was that she admired him for it. Why did this guy have to be so darn attractive?

By the time he was finished he gave her a nod and they headed back to the Land Rover.

They were certainly starting to get more relaxed around each other. Aurora took some notes from her bag. 'I checked through the computer and the diary next to Matt's desk to see if I could find out any info about the Fletchers' farm.'

She turned her head towards Eli, who was looking at her curiously. He wrinkled his nose. 'We haven't met before, have we? Because I think I would remember.'

Aurora's skin prickled. 'No,' she said as easily as she could manage.

He shook his head. 'You just seem a bit familiar.'

'I can't think how. I'm sure our paths haven't crossed.'

She could tell him. She could ask him if he'd ever watched the show. Most vets she'd come across since she'd changed profession usually said they'd tuned in to see what the show had got wrong. That didn't really surprise her. She had some friends who were nurses or medics who regularly watched some of the medical TV series to see if anything was remotely familiar.

But somehow she just couldn't get the words out. Was she embarrassed by her previous job? No. She wasn't. But it was all the repercussions from being in that show that played on her mind. It still sometimes gave her sleepless nights. The assault. The stalking.

She just didn't want to talk about all that any more. She'd put it behind her for a reason.

'Do you have a brother or sister that I might have come across?'

Darn, he was persistent.

'Only child,' she said, pasting a smile on her lips. 'I must just have one of those faces.'

She took a breath, and started on the notes again. 'I have to be honest. Matt isn't a great diary keeper.'

She held up her hand as Eli looked at her in surprise. 'Let me finish. What I mean is, the diary on his computer he didn't actually use as a diary. I think he might have started, but then he used it to just take notes, or write lists for himself. So it was almost impossible jumbling through to find out what he'd written about the Fletchers' farm.'

'Did you find anything?'

She gave a small shrug. 'Some scribbles about

further tests…phoning Dave, but I have no idea who that is. And checking symptoms.'

'Symptoms of what?'

She pulled a face. 'That's just it. He didn't write that part. It must have been all in his head.'

Eli gazed out onto the road ahead of them and pulled out. 'I just don't think I can phone Matt to ask him about this right now. I'll just have to go to the Fletchers' farm and get a feel for the place. Matt's wife texted me last night to say that his veins weren't standing up to the chemo drugs and they were putting a central line in today.'

Aurora inhaled sharply. 'So it's definitely not the time to call about work.'

'No,' he agreed, giving her a smile. 'It absolutely isn't.'

Aurora pointed to the road ahead. 'Just up on the left. This is the family that you know?'

Eli nodded. 'Well, I did when I was a kid. I mean I would have recognised them in the nearest village, but we didn't hang around together. I knew Dad was their vet, and every conversation was to do with the animals on the farm.'

'So, any clue what it might be?' she asked as he turned onto the farm road.

'Not a clue until I get there' he admitted, and she actually quite liked that about him.

When they approached, the farm seemed strangely quiet. Eli had already made his way to the nearest cow pen, but Aurora knocked on the cottage door. There were some farm vehicles around, but no actual car.

The door opened to a pink-cheeked woman. Aurora put her hand to her chest. 'I'm Aurora, the vet nurse. I'm here with Eli, our new vet. We're looking for Don Fletcher.'

The woman shook her head. 'Barb,' she said, putting her hand on her chest. 'It's taken me two weeks to persuade him to go the doctor, and his appointment is in ten minutes.' She lifted one finger to Aurora, 'Don't dare call his mobile and give him an excuse to come back.'

Aurora lifted both hands. 'I wouldn't dare. Would you mind coming and speaking to Eli?'

Barb shook her head and lifted a thick jacket from a peg near the door. She was already wearing boots so led Aurora back to where the cows were.

Eli was already checking over one cow. It was slightly scrawny-looking and in the space of time it took them to reach him he'd checked the eyes, ears and listened to the chest.

Barb held out her arms. 'Hi, Eli,' she said. 'Long time no see.' Like many farmers, she moved onto business. 'They're just generally sickly. Nothing too specific. Matt came about a month ago and said he'd come back. They're eating and drinking—maybe not as much as before. And we've been careful. It's just one herd that's affected.'

Eli stood up. 'How many herds?'

'We have beef and dairy. Three separate herds.'

'All kept in separate places?'

She nodded. 'Mainly, except for a few escape artists.'

Eli looked thoughtful and gave her a nod. 'Let's take a walk around,' he said.

They were at the farm for more than two hours. Eli looked at the layout of the fields, the dairy sheds, the pens, the hay/straw store and so much more. He examined seven different cows, all with a variety of symptoms. There were a range of coughs, some minor, some more severe, some cows were more tired than usual, and some had lost their appetite. After a long conversation, Barb agreed to keep the cows separated who were showing any symptoms, while Eli consulted about tests.

'It's a bit of a mystery,' he said as they climbed back into the Land Rover. 'None of these cows are really sick.'

'But there are enough symptoms for you to ask her to isolate?'

He nodded. 'You just never know. Lots of animals are similar to humans. Things spread. I'd like to do a bit of research and get back to the farm for more testing.' He frowned as he drove. 'I'd also like to get a chance to see Matt's notebooks to see if I can make any sense of them.'

Aurora was instantly offended. 'You mean when I couldn't?'

'If I meant that I would say it,' said Eli promptly. He continued, not giving her a chance to break in. 'I do similar things to Matt. I doodle, I write when people talk to me. And I don't always do it on the same page. If I'm writing animal notes, that's entirely different. But if I'm on the phone, and scribbling while listening, I doubt anyone would make much sense of what I've written. But it makes sense to me.'

He heaved a huge sigh, as if he knew she was still trying to make out whether to be offended or not. 'Believe me, I've driven fellow vets and nurses to despair in the past. My clinical notes are clear. But my own? Never.'

Aurora kept her mouth closed. It would be easy to pick a fight right now, but it wouldn't really serve any purpose. Today had been interesting. She'd got to see Eli Ferguson in a variety of settings, talking with a whole host of owners. He was new to most of them too, and it was fascinating watching them all try to get the measure of him, and decide if they trusted him or not.

Would she trust him with a pet? Likely. But as a person? She was still unsure.

She was certain there were sides of Eli she hadn't seen yet. He could be snappy at times— as she knew could she. His good looks were distracting. But Aurora had never been the kind of person to rely on looks alone. She always looked much deeper. And Eli's depths were still clearly hidden.

As were her own. At some point she would tell him she'd been in a TV series. It should make absolutely no difference to their working relationship, or how he saw her. But she'd sometimes felt that her previous vet colleagues had looked down on actors. Even though they shouldn't. Some of the smartest people she'd ever worked with were actors.

And whilst she could feel herself occasionally warming to Eli, she wasn't ready to reveal that part of herself. It would lead to questions, and uncomfortable memories.

And he didn't need to know that. Not yet anyway.

CHAPTER FOUR

THINGS IN THE practice settled down over the next few days. It was almost as if they fell into an easy routine, with Bert easily being the star of the show.

Aurora and Anne hadn't tried that hard to find somewhere to place him as yet. There was no urgency about the request, and he and Eli seemed suited to each other. Granted, there were occasional puddles in the hall, and even something else one day, but a vet's practice was used to animals having accidents and they all took it in their stride. It probably helped that they all frequently took Bert outside to try and imbed some toilet training rules with him.

So Aurora was surprised when Eli appeared in the doorway with a car harness for Bert. 'Will you come in the car with me? I have a potential home for Bert.'

She felt a little jolt of sadness but leaned over to grab her jacket. 'Okay, but who is it? Is it someone we'll know?'

Anne looked up from her desk. Aurora couldn't quite read the expression on her face. 'You'll know if it's the right place,' she said, looking steadily at Eli. She waited until he met her gaze, then gave him a nod. She picked up a piece of paper beside her. 'There's a message for you, Aurora. A...' she wrinkled her nose '... Fraser wants you to call him back about his cat, Arthur. The cat was recently diagnosed with diabetes. Quite insistent, actually. I did offer to speak to him, but he only wanted to speak to you.'

Aurora had an instant chill. 'They're not actually registered as our patients. And I'm sure it's the woman's name we had, not his. We saw them as an emergency.' She was silently praying that Eli would tell her not to call back.

But he was too busy with Bert. 'You can call later,' he said, not really paying attention.

Aurora gave a wave of her hand. 'Just leave it for me. I'll get to it later.' She pressed her lips together. A telephone call she could manage, but if the owner wanted to come in she would have to mention things to Anne or Eli.

As she went out to the car with Eli, she expertly manoeuvred Bert into his car harness, clipped him in, then climbed in the back seat next to him.

'What is this?' said Eli as he sat in the driver's seat.

'Last time in a car was traumatic,' said Aurora. 'I'm going to keep him company.' As Eli started the car, she continued. 'Or we're just going to sit in the back and plot against you.'

'That sounds more like it,' agreed Eli as they pulled out onto the road.

Aurora softly stroked Bert. 'So, no one has contacted the website about the picture we put up. How come you think you've found him a home?'

Eli turned his head to glance at her. 'This is just a meet and greet. I met a family the other day who said they wanted another dog. I told them we'd found a collie mix puppy who seemed healthy and they said they were interested.'

'Do you know these people? Where did you meet them? Are they patients of ours? What kind of dog do they have?'

'Whoa!' Eli laughed as he lifted one hand from the steering wheel. 'This feels like the third degree.'

'Actually, it's the fourth. I'll be telling Anne about this. If you think I'm bad…' She let her voice drift off and shook her head. 'You have absolutely no idea.'

She could see his face in the rear-view mirror. He was watching the road ahead but frowning. 'That's right. She used to give Dad a real hard time about rehoming pets.'

'And you know why that is?'

She saw the spark as the thought landed in his head. 'A dog should never be rehomed more than once.' They said it in unison and both laughed out loud.

He groaned. 'I'd forgotten about that. That's why I got the Anne stare before we left.'

'It sure is.' Aurora was smiling now as they turned into one of the nearby villages on the outskirts of Edinburgh. 'Where do they live?'

'Here, in Stockbridge. I met them at the farmers' market, and that's where they'll be today.'

Aurora sat a little straighter. 'You're not even seeing their home? We're going to the farmers' market?' She groaned. 'Give me your whole vet background again, please. Because I'm having trouble believing any of this.'

The village was already busy and it was clear the farmers' market had already started. He pulled into a car park and turned around to look at her. She'd moved Bert onto her lap and was holding him protectively.

'Do you honestly think I haven't done due diligence? I went to their house a few days ago. I met their teenage son, and their other dog. They work every day at the farmers' market, and I suggested we meet here in case the dogs aren't sure of each other. I'd hate for the other dog to be snappy because another dog came into their home.'

Aurora narrowed her gaze. She couldn't keep the ironic tone from her voice. 'You have concerns.'

Eli sighed and took a breath. 'They want a puppy to help socialise their other dog.'

'No,' said Aurora, pulling Bert closer. She was only partly joking.

'Their other dog was fine,' he said, and she was sure he was trying to sound reassuring.

'But?' she asked.

He took a breath. 'But they bought their dog at the beginning of Covid and didn't have much chance to socialise it. It's definitely a people person dog. I'm just not sure it's another dog dog.'

Aurora nodded. 'So we take Bert along, and see how the meet goes?'

The expression on his face tightened slightly. 'It's just… I won't be here for long. I don't want Bert to think he's found a home, and for me not to give him a chance of another. I like the little guy. But I will move on soon. It's selfish of me not to try when an opportunity came up.'

Aurora licked her lips. She knew it was inevitable Eli would move on. He'd said so right from the start. 'We don't seem to have any vets beating down the door.'

It was probably out of order. But she knew he'd put another advert out.

A dark look crossed his eyes but he didn't respond, just turned back around and opened the door. Aurora climbed out, clipping a lead onto Bert's collar.

The sun was rising high in the sky. Scottish summers could be unusual. It wasn't strange to have a few perfect weeks in June and then four weeks of rain for the whole of July—just when the schools closed. But today was just perfect.

She slipped her jacket off and tied it around her waist. 'It's going to be a scorcher,' she said, and turned abruptly when Eli burst out laughing.

'What?'

He shook his head. 'Your accent. It's like you have a gift for them. You sounded as though you came from Glasgow then.'

Aurora felt her cheeks flush. Accents had always been her speciality. Even though she'd stripped her own right back, with certain phrases and words, her brain seemed to automatically mimic the way she'd initially heard them used. She hadn't even thought as she'd spoken out loud.

He clearly noticed that he'd embarrassed her and pointed along the footpath. 'This way to the market. Let's have a stroll around before we go to meet the Kings.'

Aurora was grateful for the distraction and encouraged Bert as he walked well beside her. The market was busy and after a few moments' hesitation Eli bent down to pick Bert up. 'He might get overwhelmed by all the feet, and the food smells,' he said.

Aurora nodded in agreement. 'Let's go over here.'

They moved over to a large array of flowers and plants and Aurora picked some orange gerberas. 'These have always been my favourite. My gran had these in her garden when I was a child.' The seller wrapped them in some paper for her, and they moved on.

Next, they sampled some cheese. But Eli pulled a face when the one with chilli clearly hit the wrong spot. He started coughing and Aurora couldn't help but laugh, before she pulled a bottle of water from her bag. 'Stop coughing around my dog,' she murmured as he took a sip.

His eyes were watering now, and the stall-holder was laughing appreciatively. 'Always one that gets caught out,' he said with a broad smile.

They moved onto some craft stalls, bakery, bread and fish. Aurora paused for a moment. 'I wonder if I should get some for dinner.'

Eli looked at her, then licked his lips. For a second she wondered if he was nervous. 'Why don't you just let me buy you a big lunch once we've met the Kings? You might not even want a dinner.'

She looked again at the fish, wondering if she even had the ingredients in her house to make the sauce she'd want alongside. 'Okay, then. Deal,' she said.

They moved to a fruit and veg stall, where a couple in their fifties were serving and a brown cockapoo was hiding under the table.

She noticed that Eli kept Bert in his arms. 'Hi,' he greeted them, tucking Bert under one arm as he shook both their hands. 'This is Bert, the dog I told you about.'

Mrs King came out from behind the stall and started talking to Bert. 'Aren't you a wee beauty,' she said, giving his ears a rub.

Mr King came out too, and they both fussed over Bert, who seemed nonplussed by the whole event.

Mrs King eventually went to bring out their cockapoo, who was obviously shy. 'Tyler, come and meet Bert.'

Eli put Bert on the ground near Tyler, staying close. Aurora watched carefully. She'd met lots of anxious puppies and dogs. It was far more common than most people realised. Tyler was clearly one of those dogs.

There was sniffing. Bert, being a pup, was more boisterous and Tyler retreated under the table. But Mrs King persisted kindly, trying to encourage the dogs to interact. Mr King still had a few customers to serve but he was keen too, and Aurora quickly realised they were a kind couple, and true dog-lovers. She could see why Eli had considered them.

After nearly fifteen minutes, when Tyler had come out a few times, and retreated on each occasion, they finally agreed the first meeting was over. Eli shook both their hands again and picked up Bert, threading through the busy market with Aurora following.

'I know a place,' he said over his shoulder, leading her away from the main market towards a pub with multiple tables outside in the garden. There was also a little fenced-in section that was called a puppy play park, and they were right next to it.

'This place does quite a lot of fish options. Thought you might like to try, after wistfully gazing at the salmon,' he teased.

She reached over to swat his arm. 'I was not wistfully gazing at the salmon,' she said in mock horror.

'You were,' he teased, nodding at Bert. 'Wasn't she?'

It was almost as if Bert nodded too.

'Traitor,' she muttered, unable to keep the smile out of her voice. The waitress appeared, handing them menus and taking a drinks order. There were no other dogs currently in the puppy play park.

'I'll let him have a runabout,' he said as he filled up one of the water bowls. 'Let me know if anyone else appears.'

Bert was happy to play and when the waitress came back to take their food order he was jumping in and out of a stationary tyre in the play park.

She gave Eli a stare as she ordered. 'I'll have the sea bream, please.'

He raised his eyebrows as he handed his menu back to the waitress. 'I'll have the Cajun salmon,' he said sheepishly, and they both laughed as the waitress laughed.

The sun was beating down, although their table was a little shaded by a parasol. Aurora automatically took some sunscreen out of her bag and put some on her arms, before handing it over to Eli. 'Danger of being a redhead,' she said with a smile. 'Always have sunscreen.'

Eli nodded gratefully as he slid some on too. 'What did you think of the meet?' he asked.

'I think it's a no,' she said simply, holding up her diet Coke towards him. 'Tyler isn't ready for another dog in the house. He's too shy, and I think there might be a good chance he'll retreat further into himself.'

Eli tipped his head to one side and looked at her curiously. After a second he lifted his soda and blackcurrant too. 'I completely agree.'

'What will you tell the Kings?' she asked curiously.

He looked thoughtful for a moment. 'They adore Tyler,' he said. 'I think they'll know themselves. They would never do anything to upset him.'

'Here's hoping,' she said, glancing over at Bert. 'Oh, look, he's got the zoomies.'

They laughed as they watched Bert run around in circles at a hundred miles an hour.

'Do you have any other visits today?' she asked.

He shook his head. 'I'm going to do some more reading about cows,' he said with a sigh. 'Something is definitely bothering me.'

'It'll come to you,' said Aurora with a smile as her sea bream was put down in front of her. 'Usually in the middle of the night, and completely out of nowhere.'

Eli looked a bit surprised. 'Is that when things come to you?'

'Always,' she said as she sampled her fish. 'Like, if I've met someone that day but can't place them. And it annoys me all day. Then, in the middle of the night, I'll remember it was Sally from school's Auntie Jean. Or it was a patient from Hawkshead who has moved miles away, and because I'm not there any more I couldn't place them.'

'Do you ever sleep?' he asked with a smile on his face.

A memory flitted across her brain, and she pushed it to one side. Sleep at one time had evaded her for months.

She gave him a smile. 'I sleep like a log. It's the one reason I've got a cat and not a dog.'

Eli looked momentarily confused. She waved one hand. 'Because at the beginning you have to get up with a puppy in the middle of the night. Them waking because they need the toilet would generally wake a person. But…' she sighed '… I have slept through an alarm in the middle of the night before. Cats can use a litter tray. Not useful if you're trying to toilet train a puppy.'

'Where were you going that you needed an alarm in the middle of the night?'

It was a natural question, but it made her stall. She'd been going to catch a flight at Heathrow for filming in South Africa. She'd ended up with a taxi driver hammering on her door to wake her. But she just didn't want to get those words out. 'I was going to a festival,' were the words that came out. From nowhere, from absolutely nowhere, and she was cringing before she'd finished the sentence.

'Do you like festivals?' Eli asked, his eyes brightening. 'Where have you been? I love festivals. Used to do them all when I was a bit younger.' He gave her a broad grin. 'Remember the famous year at Glastonbury when it turned into a mud bath? That was me.'

Her brain was now on overdrive and it was entirely her own doing. 'Isle of Man,' she said as a little bit of her died inside at the continuation of her work of fiction.

His brow furrowed for a second. 'What one was that?'

'Can't remember,' she said quickly. 'I just realised sleeping in a tent was not for me.'

'Not a camper?'

She shook her head. At least this was true. 'Not a chance. I like comfort. I like electricity. I like heating. I want a comfy bed. A kettle. And the last thing I want to do in this world is have to squat in a forest to pee.'

He started laughing again, and Aurora started to relax. 'You're a five-star hotel girl, then?'

She held up her glass to him again. 'Without a shadow of a doubt.'

Part of her was a little sorry. If she'd been honest about her previous job, she could have told him about the wonderful lodges she'd stayed in while they were filming the vet series in South Africa. The lodges were in the middle of the

Kruger National Park and were amazing. She could have been honest about the animals and wonderful vets. But again, it would lead to memories of the not good parts. The assault. The stalking. She'd worked so hard to put all that behind her. The spider-sense feeling had led her to have another online session with her counsellor the other day, and she was taking comfort from some of the outputs of the session. There was no quick fix. Not for what she'd gone through.

She just didn't want to let those memories in, not on a gorgeous sunny day like this. Not when she was currently watching Bert jump around a dog play park having the time of his life.

It hadn't gone the way he'd wanted. But, then again, Eli wasn't entirely sure how he'd wanted it to go. He'd meant it entirely when he'd said he wanted to give Bert the chance of a good and permanent home. But it had felt too easy to say that the Kings wouldn't be a good fit.

He could feel himself becoming even more curious about Aurora. There was that familiar feeling around her. Anne had mentioned casually that there was no other half in her life. The more he spent time with her, the more the walls he'd built up around himself seemed to relax a little. Or maybe it was the setting. Being back at his father's practice hadn't been quite as bad as he'd thought it might. The work was interesting.

But he still worried about trusting those around him. It was ridiculous. He wasn't responsible for the accounts at the practice. That was still Matt's domain. But whilst he was off sick Matt had given him access to the practice credit cards, and told him that 'one of the girls' would likely handle the salaries.

It made him naturally jumpy. He wasn't sure how things normally worked around here. Last thing he wanted to do was interfere with the normal. But didn't he also have a responsibility to keep an eye on things? He couldn't deny he still had trust issues when it came to money— and especially for the business. He'd already let one business go to the wall; he couldn't let it happen to another. He pushed the money aspect from his head.

Because Aurora had hit a nerve earlier. He'd only had one enquiry so far about joining the practice—and it was from someone who wouldn't qualify for another six months. Eli spent his nights scouring the internet for other vet jobs— so why would he imagine anyone else wouldn't do the same? Did the outskirts of Edinburgh compare to the heat of San Diego, or the learning curve of working in the bush in Australia?

Bert gave a short yap—not quite a bark yet—and Eli turned his attention back to their puppy.

The thought stopped him hard. *Their* puppy? The practice's puppy, of course. He gave a little shudder.

'Cold?' asked Aurora innocently. Her dark red hair had fanned around her shoulders, and he could see her attracting glances. He was trying so hard not to notice just how attractive she was, or how the casual drift of her perfume instantly caught his attention.

Had he learned nothing from his last experience?

He set down his knife and fork. 'Not at all,' he said quickly. 'Want another drink?'

Aurora shook her head and nodded behind him. 'I think there's another dog about to come in.'

Eli caught sight of the black Labrador entering the pub grounds with her owners. He picked up Bert from the play park and slipped him back on the lead next to them. 'I'll just settle the bill,' he said, signalling to the waitress. 'Is there anywhere else you'd like to go?'

Aurora leaned back a little, stretching out her back and looking thoughtful. 'There was a bookshop along the street. It had stacked tables outside. I wouldn't mind having a look.'

'Sure,' said Eli, scanning his card to the machine the waitress brought over. 'It's a bit less busy down there. Let's see how Bert does.'

They walked casually down the picturesque street. There was no traffic as this part of the road was cobbled. All the shops had old-fashioned frontages, painted in a variety of colours. Some had window boxes on the upper floors filled with colourful flowers.

'This place is like a picture postcard,' murmured Aurora as she walked alongside him.

'It's a lovely town,' said Eli, stopping and looking through the glass of the butcher's shop.

After a few moments Aurora bent closer, her hair brushing against his face as she joked, 'Eli Ferguson, are you wistfully gazing at a steak?'

He burst out laughing and shook his head as he walked away. Two minutes later, Aurora stopped walking as she stared in the front window of a clothing shop.

She held up one hand as he opened his mouth. 'Yes, Eli Ferguson, I'm wistfully gazing at a pink shirt.' Her hand went to her back. 'In fact, give me two minutes.'

Eli watched in amazement as she ducked inside, had a conversation with the woman behind the till, who crossed to the other side of the shop and looked through a few hanging shirts before pulling out a pink one and carrying it back to the counter. Aurora leaned over to look at the tag and nodded in agreement as she pulled out her purse.

Literally, two minutes later, she was back by his side, bag in hand.

'You just bought that.'

'I did.' Her smile reached right across her face. It was the first time he'd noticed her eyes sparkle. She clicked her fingers. 'This is the way I shop. I see something, I like it. I check my size and I buy it.' She shrugged and laughed. 'Boyfriends in the past have loved it, but my girlfriends all hate it. They like to spend hours in shops.'

'You don't need to try things on?'

She wrinkled her brow. 'I know what size I am. Unless the shop is unusual and runs bigger or smaller than normal, it's never an issue. And the people behind the counter know that about their clothes. They do generally let me know.' She smiled and held up her shirt. 'Fastest female shopper ever?'

He gave a short laugh. 'I'm sure there must be some kind of medal for that.'

She rolled her eyes. 'Guess what? That medal is made of either books or chocolate.'

In a lightning move, Aurora ducked into the next shop, a bakers, and came out carrying a white box. 'Don't ask—' she smiled '—it's a surprise for the journey home.'

They moved to the next shop, which was stacked up with books on the tables outside. People were browsing casually. 'Why don't you go in?' said Eli. 'Bert and I will wait outside.'

She shook her head. 'Oh, no. I love to rummage. The best and most obscure stuff is likely to be out here.' She started sifting through the stacks and Eli joined her. It only took a second for him to see something that interested him. He pulled out a dog-eared hardback with a faded blue cover.

She moved closer. 'What is it?'

He flicked it open. 'Just a book about an old shipwreck.' He gave a rueful smile. 'This is my weakness.'

She looked at him with a broad smile. 'Not old musty vet books?'

He had the tiniest inkling of something again. But he pushed it away. 'Oh, no, that was my father's weakness. I spent my life surrounded by them, and inherited most of them.' He held up the book. 'Shipwrecks is my go-to non-fiction.'

'Egypt is mine,' she countered, and he couldn't help but be intrigued.

'Really? Why?'

'So much history, so much unexplained, so many interesting people. And how did they build those pyramids?'

He smiled. 'You don't go for the conspiracy theories?'

Her eyebrows raised. 'Oh, I love those. I half believe that thirty-year-old film about gates made of stars that said the aliens brought the pyramids down and they are secretly space-ships.'

'That would be kind of cool.' He held her green gaze. She studied him in return, and for a few seconds he was frozen. Stuck in that place that made the sounds and colours fade around them, and for Aurora to become his only focus. She was captivating. Her perfume aroma drifted near to him on the breeze, sparking his senses. For a moment there was nothing else. Just her, and him. He could already imagine her in that pink shirt she'd just bought, and how it would bring out the red in her hair even more vividly.

And then a little body nudged against his leg and broke him out of his momentary spell.

He blinked and shook his head, licking his lips. 'Think there's any Egypt in amongst this lot?' He nodded to the stacks of books.

'Give me a minute,' she said, and he watched as she took a few steps, her eyes scanning up and down the books like a true shopping pro-fessional, moving a few stacks before stepping back with a sigh. 'Nope, no Egypt.'

'You did that in under a minute.'

'Told you. I don't waste time.'

'Want to go inside?'

She glanced down at Bert, who had tucked himself under the table. 'Let me go and grab a thriller. I need something to read tonight. I'll pay for yours too.'

She went to add something, but Eli held up one hand, laughing, 'You'll only be a minute.'

True to form, she came back out holding a new release. 'Set on a cruise ship,' she said with a grin. 'A woman wakes up and everyone else is gone.'

'That does sound good,' said Eli. 'I might borrow it when you're done.' He held up the book she'd bought him. 'Tell me how much I owe you.'

'Don't be silly,' she said. 'You bought lunch.'

'Then thank you.' He looked down at Bert. 'Come on, little guy, that's enough walking for today.'

Bert seemed quite happy to continue, but the heat was building and Eli didn't want to walk him on the pavements any longer than necessary. He bent down and picked him up, tucking him under one arm.

Aurora leaned over and stroked Bert's head. 'We're going to find someone for you, little guy, don't worry.'

'Have you ever had a dog before?' He was curious.

She nodded. 'Yes, and no. My parents bought a red Labrador when I was a kid, but couldn't handle it. My gran ended up taking Max and since I went there after school every day I was always with him.'

'So, it worked out well?'

'It did. He was a great dog, and my gran was just too old to handle a puppy again when he finally passed away. It leaves such a gap in your life—you know, when you lose an animal.'

He looked at her carefully as they reached the car. 'So, if you could bring your dog to work every day, would you think about it?'

Her steps slowed. 'What do you mean?'

He opened one door to strap Bert in. 'I mean, I've fixed up the kennels outside now. Bert is quite happy running around in the enclosure during the day.'

'You want me to take Bert?'

He was trying to find a delicate way to put this, but was clearly failing. 'Well, maybe.'

'But what about in winter? There's no way I'd leave a dog outside in the snow we get.' She climbed into the car, but kept talking. 'And what about when you leave and there's a new partner? They might not take kindly to staff bringing their pets to work.'

'Or they might love the idea.'

She pulled a face. 'Not when we have to go

into emergency surgery and might be stuck in there for hours.'

Eli sighed and nodded. 'Okay, so you've got me there. But if that happens in the next few weeks, Bert will need to go in the kennels out back. At least I know he's safe there. It was just a thought,' he said as he started the car.

He pulled out into the traffic and Aurora opened the white box. 'Iced raspberry doughnuts,' she said, offering him one.

'These match your new shirt,' he said as he took a bite.

'So they do.' She smiled as she took a bite of her own. 'I didn't even think of that.'

As they pulled out of the village and onto the country road he shot her a glance again. 'At least tell me you'll think about it.'

She gave him a hard stare. 'About Bert?'

He nodded.

'What if you decide you want to keep him yourself and take him wherever you decide to go?'

Eli shot a glance in his rear-view mirror at the puppy sleeping on the back seat. 'It would get too complicated,' he said. 'Particularly if I decide to go abroad again.'

'You're not done running away yet?' she asked.

The words prickled, and his hands tensed on the wheel. 'I'm not running.'

'Okay,' she said simply as he shot her a sideways glance. But the expression on her face made it clear she didn't believe him. 'But why would your next job be far away again?'

He swallowed. He could tell her the truth. He could say he'd opened up a practice for the last few years in England, and ended up going bankrupt because he'd been conned. But somehow, telling that story didn't have a huge amount of appeal.

'You could always just stay a bit longer at your dad's old practice,' she said, as if it were the easiest thing in the world. 'Or stay for good.'

It was like throwing a bucket of water over him. 'I won't be staying,' he said firmly.

Aurora opened her mouth again. It was clear she had a million arguments around this. But she must have caught sight of the expression on his face because, instead of speaking, she gave half an eye-roll and took another bite of her doughnut.

He glanced at his own expression in the mirror. It wasn't pretty. His jaw was clenched tight, just like his hands on the wheel, and his own doughnut was currently languishing in his lap.

He took a breath and let his shoulders relax. This had been a good day. Probably the first he'd had in a long time.

He wasn't going to let anything spoil it.

'Just promise you'll think about it,' he said again.

A hint of a smile appeared on her lips. 'You're going to get my new boss to sack me, aren't you?'

He winked. 'Don't worry, we'll write it into your contract that you can bring your pets to work.'

Aurora sighed and leaned back in her seat, 'Okay, I'll think about it.' She wagged her finger at him. 'But that's all. *Think* about it.'

And as the countryside sped past, Eli smiled too.

CHAPTER FIVE

AURORA WASN'T TOO sure how to feel about anything.

Her afternoon with Eli Ferguson had whipped up a whole host of strange feelings. She hadn't expected to enjoy herself so much. She liked sparring with Eli. She liked finding out more about him.

And she couldn't pretend she wasn't a little disappointed when he'd said, categorically, that he wouldn't be staying at his father's practice. There had been a definite edge to his tone. One that made her understand there was likely a whole host of things she didn't know about.

Anne hadn't been too free with information. It was obvious she had a deep loyalty to David Ferguson and, in turn, to his son.

As for Bert? She'd love a dog. But, due to the nature of her job, it just wasn't practical. If Eli had actually meant what he'd said...

The phone rang and she answered automatically. 'Ferguson and Green veterinary practice.'

'Can I speak to Aurora, please?'

There was something about the voice. It instantly made her defensive.

She was hesitant with her reply. 'Who is calling, please?'

'It's Fraser, Fraser Dobbs. She was supposed to phone me back about our cat, Arthur.'

Aurora straightened up at the implication. 'You were called back, Mr Dobbs. A message was left for you yesterday at four-twenty p.m.' She could remember precisely when she'd called because she'd been relieved to get an answer machine.

There was a humph noise at the end of the line. Another thing that pressed her dislike buttons.

'Well, I want to speak to her now.'

'You are speaking to her, Mr Dobbs.'

He went into an immediate tirade about the cat, and how essential it was for him to come and see Aurora, and when could he get an appointment. She tried not to let her past experiences affect her. Maybe this gentleman was just concerned about his animal, and wasn't coping with the long-term condition.

She asked some questions, explaining things as best as she could. But everything always came back to the same thing—he wanted to bring Arthur in, and see her.

It made Aurora distinctly uncomfortable.

It wasn't entirely uncommon for some patients to prefer to see the same individual in a vet practice. It helped with continuity of care, and with maintaining therapeutic relationships. Occasionally, some pet owners became a little possessive over staff members, but this was usually when a pet was severely ill.

Aurora looked at the appointment calendar. Her spider-sense was tingling again, and while she wouldn't refuse to see a patient, she would make certain she wasn't going to be in the practice alone.

She asked a few questions around his partner, to see if she would be attending too, letting him know it was best to see them together, in case his partner had any questions of her own. He made some brush-off excuse to let her know that he would be attending alone, and that his partner didn't really understand anything about it.

After another few minutes they agreed on an appointment the following week, when Aurora knew that Eli would be around. She would talk to him about this later.

She replaced the handset, wondering what on earth she would say to him about this. As an employee, she should let him know that the individual made her uncomfortable. But, on the other hand, she didn't want him to think that she was unwilling to work with difficult clients, or when a pet owner had anxiety over their condition.

Bert trotted around the corner towards her, and she bent automatically to rub him behind the ears.

'Naughty, naughty,' came the sigh from the corridor.

'What?' Aurora looked up, amused, and surprised, with her eyes wide.

Eli had a cloth in his hand as he rounded the corner. He almost fell over them.

'Oops,' he said. Then his face coloured.

'Bert,' he said quickly, 'I was talking to Bert.'

Aurora glanced down the corridor, where a small puddle glinted in the sunlight. 'Really?' she teased. 'Because I'm not sure you're allowed to talk to employees that way.'

She picked up Bert and stood up, walking into the nearby consulting room.

'And doesn't our good vet know that our dogs don't get into trouble when they pee indoors? We just take them outside and clean it up without a fuss.'

'Well, this will be non-fuss number four this morning,' said Eli as he grabbed the mop and bucket from the corner.

She looked at Bert. 'Come on, son. Let's go outside for a bit.'

She left Eli mopping as she took Bert out to

the run next to the kennels and set him down. Almost immediately, he did another pee. 'Good boy,' she said as she gave him a tiny treat.

'He does it to play me,' sighed Eli behind her. 'He pees inside, I bring him out. He pees outside, I praise him, take him back outside and he looks me in the eye, and does another.'

'Have you forgotten how hard the puppy stage is?' She smiled.

'Oh, I think you could say that.'

'When was the last time you had one?'

He shook his head. 'Honestly? Years ago. I've adopted or rescued mainly.'

'The old boys and girls?'

He nodded. It was common practice that vets or shelters were frequently left elderly pets, particularly when costs became more difficult for owners. Older dogs and cats in shelters were often overlooked when people came to find a new pet.

'There's something nice about giving an old dog or cat a great last few years,' said Eli, a wistful look on his face. 'Sometimes it's only a few months, but just devoting yourself to their care and attention for that period of time, letting them know they're settled and loved, is worth it.'

Aurora straightened in surprise. 'Eli Ferguson. You almost sound as if you have a big melting heart.'

'With animals?' he said. 'Every. Single. Time.'

'And with people?' She couldn't help herself, and as he turned to look at her she had a wide smile on her face.

He wrinkled his brow and looked a bit sorry about life. 'When you're concentrating on your animals there isn't much time for people,' was how he answered the question.

But Aurora wasn't going to let him get away with that. 'Come on, you mean to tell me that in all the time you stayed in—' she swiped her hand '—Florida, Spain, France and Maine, you never dated?'

He raised his eyebrows and the edges of his mouth tilted up in amusement, 'Good memory.'

'I'm a stickler for details. You'll learn that.'

He was still amused. 'Will I?'

'Only if you answer the question.'

It was like a standoff, but Eli was too quick. 'I will if you will.'

She tilted her head and put her hands on her hips. 'What?'

'Your other half? Or exes? You haven't mentioned anyone.'

There were a few seconds of silence.

'You first,' said Aurora.

Eli licked his lips. 'I dated a few people casually in each of the places you mentioned.' He took a slow breath, and then said rather slowly,

'I've kind of learned I shouldn't mix my personal and professional life.'

Wow. That was saying something. It was like a slap on the face. And though her first thought was to be offended—particularly when this had definitely seemed a bit flirtatious—she kind of got the impression there was more to this. Eli Ferguson actually looked a bit hurt, and a bit wary.

And he would never realise this, but his words actually resonated with her.

'I dated someone at work once, and it didn't work out particularly well.'

'Really?'

She wrinkled her nose. 'I was a bit younger, and it was just kind of awkward, when you split up and still have to work together.'

He let out a long, slow breath, along with a kind of ironic laugh. 'You have no idea,' he said.

She stared at him, curious. 'Well, that's kind of cryptic.'

He paused for a moment, as if he was actually going to give her more information—fill in some of the blanks that she was conscious were still there. But he just put his hands on his hips and stretched his back. 'That's for another time, and likely a lot of beer.'

She blinked and pressed her lips together, because she hated where her head had automatically gone. Straight back to the pub they'd had lunch in, but there at night, on an actual date. Her brain did that in a few milliseconds, and she was cursing it.

She didn't want to think about Eli Ferguson like that. One, he was her temporary boss. Two, he wasn't staying. Three, there were still some things he wasn't sharing. And four, she hadn't been honest with him about herself. None of these things could add up to a healthy fling or relationship.

She gave an amused smile.

'What is it?' he asked.

She shook her head. 'Daft memories. Mainly around a very bad date and falling into a table full of beer that, unfortunately, was all in pint glasses instead of bottles.'

He shuddered. 'Messy.' Then one eyebrow arched. 'But was it you that fell on it, or your date?'

'Oh, it was my date. He was a friend of a friend, and had gone to the pub early as he was nervous and drank himself blind drunk. When I arrived, he got up to buy me a drink and went straight back down again.' She bit her bottom lip to stop herself from smiling too hard.

'Poor guy probably never recovered.'

'Oh, he did. I danced at his wedding last year. You know the mutual friend? They got married.'

'She set you up when she liked him herself?'

Aurora smiled. '*He* set me up. One of the best weddings I've ever been to, and the part about the almost date made it into the wedding speech.'

Bert had finished his toileting and made a beeline for them both, catapulting himself at Eli, who had to reach out his hands to catch him. 'Whoa, little guy.' He held him up to his face. 'How can someone so small jump so high?'

The phone started ringing inside and Aurora darted in to answer it. Eli followed her in, carrying Bert. She gave him a careful look as she spoke on the phone. 'Hey, Marianne, how is Matt? He is? Okay…' She paused. 'Yes, I'm here with Eli now.' She mouthed the word to him. *Visit?*

He immediately nodded.

'Yes, we'd love to. Today?'

Eli nodded again.

'No problem, we'll see you in an hour.' And then she paused for a moment. 'Is there anything you need? Anything you want us to bring?'

Marianne started to immediately say no, then there was a small noise at the end of the phone, and Aurora knew she was crying.

'Marianne, ask me for anything. It's absolutely no bother and we're happy to do it.' There were a few more sniffles and something about not wanting to be a bother. 'You're not a bother. Send me a wee text, and we'll pick up whatever you need on the way there.'

'Everything okay?' asked Eli as she replaced the receiver.

Aurora shook her head. 'She phoned because Matt's concerned he didn't get to do a proper handover and wants to see you.' She gave a sad smile. 'He's conscious that not all his notes are up-to-date.'

Eli pulled a face. 'His notebook—I haven't even had a chance to look at that yet. Where is it?'

'In your desk drawer,' she said, not taking pleasure in the fact he hadn't looked yet. She'd begun to actually wonder if she might have missed something he could spot.

He opened his drawer, pulled out an A5 green-covered notebook and started flicking. His smile was broad. 'Matt is exactly the same scrawler and doodler as I am.'

Aurora watched him as her phone sounded with a text message notification. 'Marianne said that he's sleeping loads right now while he's mid-treatment, so might not be awake for too long.' She gave a soft smile. 'She's also given me a list of girl's things that she needs. She's clearly been running about for Matt and forgot about herself.'

She looked out of the window as Eli kept flicking, writing a few random notes himself. 'I wonder…' Her voice tailed off.

'You wonder what?' His blue eyes met hers.

She pulled a face. 'It's just that on the way there we'll pass their favourite restaurant. I've been there with them a few times. I know what they like.' She glanced at her watch. 'It's nearly five o'clock. How do you feel about us getting them some takeout dinner?'

'Sounds like a great idea.' He glanced down again and his hand froze over a word. 'Oh, no!' He let out a sharp expression.

'What?' Aurora was genuinely startled. She moved behind him to bend over his shoulder and see the word that had stopped him.

Badger. With a question mark next to it.

It was on the bottom corner of one page. The corner had creased upwards so it was almost hidden. But the top of the page held information about the Fletchers' farm.

Eli closed his eyes for a second. 'Don't suppose we know the last time the Fletchers' cattle had their TB tests?'

Aurora instantly felt her mouth go dry. Bovine TB was serious. Herds could be wiped out. Farms could be ruined. Badgers were a protected species, but could also have TB and carry it, and secrete it in their urine, faeces or any wounds. If cattle had direct contact with infected badgers, or if cattle feed or water was contaminated by badger excretions, then TB could pass between the species.

'Is that what Matt suspected?'

Eli flicked another few pages. 'It could be. It's not clear. The symptoms could match, but it could also be a host of other things. Darn it.'

'Maybe that's what Matt wants to talk to you about?'

He nodded solemnly. 'Could be.' He looked up again. 'Do you want to get changed before we go visiting? And, apart from the restaurant, where do we need to stop off?'

'A supermarket,' she said quickly. 'And yes, I will get changed. Is it okay to use the shower upstairs?'

'Of course,' he said, settling back down at the computer to keep checking some files.

By the time Aurora came down the stairs she'd changed into the pink shirt she'd bought the other day and jeans, and her hair was combed loose. Eli had made a few notes with questions to ask Matt, but he was also conscious his father's old partner might not be up to it. He'd dashed upstairs to change his shirt and brush his hair and was ready to go. He hadn't been sure of what Matt's relationship had been like with the newest member of staff, because there hadn't been an opportunity to have that conversation, but from

Aurora's expression on the phone today it was clear she was close to both Matt and Marianne.

Her suggestion of buying them dinner from their favourite restaurant was thoughtful and a nice touch.

The drive was just over half an hour, and whilst thoughts of TB were flitting around his head he tried to push them away.

'Didn't take you long to wear your new shirt,' he said.

Aurora looked down at herself and brushed the shirt. 'This is actually the second time. It's soft and really comfortable. I might go back and try and get it in another colour.'

He smiled, doing his best not to notice how good it looked on her. Her dark red hair was stunning against the pastel pink of the shirt, and it seemed to complement and enhance the green of her eyes. His eyes couldn't help but linger on her lips. Her make-up was always light, but she'd clearly put on some extra lipstick when getting ready. That, with her long lashes, made her look like some kind of film star.

He had a weird jolt again. Just like he'd had before around her. The wave of strange familiarity that he just couldn't put his finger on.

They chatted easily about books, films and a few of the farms along the way. Eli started telling her about cases Matt and his father had dealt with when he was a boy. It was odd how easily the memories flowed. But these ones weren't dimmed by feelings of neglect. When anything had been happening in the practice, his father had welcomed any interest or assistance.

'The stoat ended up where?' laughed Aurora, tears streaming down her face.

'In our pipes. First under the floorboards in the staff kitchen. Then inside the wall upstairs. He was like a magical Houdini. It took seven days to finally catch him again.'

'What did his owner say?'

'Oh—' Eli waved his hand '—that was old Gus Bryant. He just laughed and said to bring him back when we found him.'

They pulled up outside the supermarket and Eli joined Aurora inside. She hovered near the tower of baskets, then changed her mind and grabbed a trolley. 'You know what. I'm just going to buy them some things. Food, household stuff, toiletries.'

'I'll grab some crime books,' said Eli. 'Matt always loved those.'

Aurora didn't scrimp. She bought chicken, fish, steaks, some fresh fruit and vegetables, alongside milk, cheese, crusty bread, and a whole array of women's toiletries. As they neared the checkout she stopped at the chocolate aisle and ran her eye along it. 'There!' she said happily.

'Marianne's favourites.' They packed the food into the boot of his car and she directed him to the local restaurant.

Eli couldn't help but look at the menu as Aurora ordered Matt and Marianne's favourites. He put his hand on her arm. 'Once we've seen Matt, we'll come back and eat here. We might as well. No point driving back and making food at home.'

For a second she didn't say anything, and he realised his hand was still on her arm and she was staring at it.

'Sorry,' he said instantly, pulling his hand away.

'It's fine,' she said briskly, but he noticed her rub the spot with her other hand.

It only took five minutes for the kitchen to put the meals together, and Aurora carried them in covered plates. As they pulled up outside Matt's house, Eli felt a wave of nerves. He had spoken to Matt on numerous occasions, but he hadn't actually seen him in person since his father's funeral.

Everything about the house was familiar, from the six grey steps leading up to the pale blue door to the front window that spilled out warm light. He got the shopping from the boot as Aurora climbed the steps, balancing the plates and ringing the bell.

The familiar ringtone of the ancient bell made

his face break into a smile. A few seconds later, Marianne opened the door and ushered them both inside. Her eyes filled with tears when Aurora explained what they'd brought.

'You're an angel,' she said, sweeping Aurora into a careful hug, then taking the plates from her. 'Let me put them in the oven to stay warm. Matt's just taken his anti-sickness meds, and we need to give them time to work.'

'He's not keeping things down?' asked Eli, concern lacing his voice.

The small, grey-haired woman met his gaze. It was almost as if she hadn't heard what he'd said. 'So like your father,' she said with a smile, before holding him in a long hug.

His awkwardness vanished in an instant, with the familiar smells of the house, and warmth from Marianne. 'I've missed you both,' he said quietly. She would know. She would know exactly what he meant, and how he felt, because Marianne had been witness to it all. She was too kind to ever say a bad word about her friend— his father—but that didn't mean she'd been blind to his shortcomings.

They padded quietly through to the sitting room. Even though it was a warm summer evening, the fire was lit and Matt was covered in a dark red blanket. His treatment was obviously making him feel the cold.

His skin was translucent, and he'd lost a lot of weight since the last time Eli had seen him. He was shocked by Matt's appearance. But Aurora didn't miss a beat, she crossed the room in a few steps and dropped a kiss on Matt's cheek.

'It's so good to see you. We're missing you so much.' She quickly mentioned a list of patients who'd enquired after him and wanted him to come back soon.

Warmth spread through Eli's chest. This was the benefit of being a long-term vet somewhere. The patients and people knew you. They noticed when you weren't there. Had anyone noticed when Eli had left any of his previous posts?

He hoped so, but it wouldn't be the same as this. He moved quickly, first shaking Matt's hand, then kissing his cheek too, and automatically sitting on the little footstool at the bottom of the chair.

Matt bent forward and cupped his cheek. 'It's so good to see you again.'

Eli's hand covered Matt's. He had so many good memories of this couple. So many times he'd stayed at their house, or had their support for school or sports events.

'You too,' he said slowly, hoping his voice wouldn't break.

There was a chance he wasn't going to have Matt much longer. He didn't need to ask questions. He didn't need to focus on scans or treatment plans. One look at Matt, plus the expression on Marianne's face at the door, told him everything he needed to know.

They didn't have children of their own. Marianne had nieces and nephews, but Eli had been the one to whom they'd shown undying support.

He settled on the stool as Matt started talking about the practice. It was clear he wanted to get things in order. As Eli pulled Matt's notebook from his back pocket he wished this didn't need to happen. But he had to respect Matt's wishes.

Aurora caught his eye and nodded towards the kitchen. 'I'm going to help Marianne unpack,' she said.

Matt quickly went through some patients, including a planned complicated surgery that Eli would have the skills to take over.

'What about the Fletchers' farm?' he asked cautiously.

But Matt was still sharp as a tack. 'Cows still sick?'

Eli nodded. 'I found some of your notes, but they weren't exactly in order.'

'It's the badgers,' said Matt without hesitation. 'Check the badgers.' Then, as if he could read Eli's mind, 'The bovine TB testing is due next month.'

Eli's heart dropped like a stone. He'd half

hoped it had recently been scheduled and bovine TB could have been ruled out. But not now. 'I'll deal with it,' he said quietly.

Matt looked as if he wanted to say a whole lot more, but sagged back against the cushions on his armchair. 'Okay,' he replied simply.

He glanced to the door and back to Eli. 'So, you've put all that stuff behind you?'

Eli knew exactly what he was referring to. He sighed. 'It's resulted in bankruptcy. Iona will face criminal charges if she's ever found, but the practice property was repossessed and I was left with a whole pile of debts.'

'The staff?'

'I used my savings to pay their salaries. I did that as soon as I realised what had happened, and knew there was much more to come. So, I prioritised their salaries and notice periods, gave them all references, and closed the practice doors while the fallout happened.'

'You could have come to me!'

'For my stupidity? For trusting someone who took my livelihood? She got enough from me. I would never have come to you for something like that. It was my mess. I had to sort it.'

'I would have helped you,' Matt said shakily, and Eli's heart squeezed inside his chest.

'I know you would have. But I can start again. I just need to sort things out with yours and

Dad's place, and then I'll take myself off somewhere else, and decide what comes next.'

'You have a practice. You have staff. You have
a community where some people have known
you since you were a boy.'

Eli couldn't get a reply out. He wouldn't hurt
this man for the world. He couldn't explain how
the practice brought back memories he found
hard to push away. He just gave a shake of his
head. 'I just can't do it. Not now.'

Matt tilted his head a little as laughter could
be heard from the kitchen. 'What do you think
of Aurora?'

Eli gave an embarrassed laugh. 'We've exchanged a few words, but she seems to be a good
vet nurse.'

'She is. Smart as a whip. I'm worried someone will try to steal her. When she started I had
a few emails from another vet who had met her
down at Hawkshead. They were impressed by
her. I think a few had given her alternative of-
fers, but…' he smiled broadly '…she chose us.'

Eli was curious about that. 'She's young to
move up here by herself. Does she have family
around here?'

Matt shook his head. 'She's from Liverpool.
No family up here. As far as I'm aware, her mum
and dad are still in Liverpool.'

Liverpool. He was getting used to hearing the remnants of the accent when it emerged.

'No husband?' Eli queried.

Matt leaned forward. He had a grin on his face, and a sparkle in his eyes. This. This was the way he'd always remembered Matt. 'And why would you be asking that? Has Aurora Hendricks caught your eye, Elijah?'

Eli gave a fake shudder. 'Don't. You only call me Elijah when things are serious.'

'And they are. She's a beautiful girl, with a big heart and…' he narrowed his gaze on Eli '…possibly too good for you,' he finished with undisguised relish.

Eli laughed. Matt had always teased him like this. All good-heartedly.

He glanced at the open doorway again. 'She's…nice,' he said. 'Thoughtful. And passionate about the animals.'

There was a noise and they both looked up. Marianne was carrying in the steaming hot plates of food on a tray. The smell was delicious. 'Look what Aurora and Eli brought us from Eldershaw's restaurant. Our favourite.'

Eli stood up, pulling over the nearby table so Matt's food could be close to him. He leaned over again and kissed Matt on the cheek. 'It was lovely to see you—enjoy your dinner and we'll catch up in a few days.'

Matt's frail hand caught his and squeezed it hard. 'Love you, Eli,' he said with a glimmer of a tear in his eye.

'You too,' was as much as Eli could manage, before hugging and kissing Marianne too, then heading to the door.

When they got outside, they both stood on the top step for a few moments. He could hear Aurora's shaky breaths; his own weren't much better.

'Okay?' he asked.

'I could really use dinner about now,' she answered.

He was grateful. Neither of them wanted to admit how sick Matt was. There was time for that later.

They climbed down the steps, into the car and drove back to the restaurant, where they were seated at a table at a window looking out over the back terrace and gardens. The sun was just beginning to dim, sending streaks of orange and red across the darkening sky.

'Do you want me to drive back?' she asked as they looked at their menus.

'Why would you ask that?'

Her eyes shone with sympathy. 'Because you've known Matt all your life. I saw the shock register on your face when you saw him. I just figured you might like to sit here and have a beer with your dinner.'

He was struck by how considerate she was being. 'I've driven the car before on visits to farms, so I know I'm covered on the insurance,' she added.

He hadn't even thought of that. Thank goodness she had. 'You know, I'd really appreciate that,' he said.

Eli's head was all over the place. The swamping memories, being back at his dad's practice. The mixed emotions of the love he still felt for his father, added to the adult perspective now, where he could see he'd been neglected in some ways. The anger that still simmered on a daily basis at being conned so thoroughly, and so well, that his only option had been to use his savings to pay the staff wages before declaring bankruptcy. That deep down regret that he'd lost the ability to trust people, and it now affected his everyday life.

And yet he looked at Aurora and felt…something.

He didn't want to, and he shouldn't. But he couldn't help it. Something just seemed to radiate between them, to spark. Whether it was the too-long glances or the occasional flirtatious chat, he wasn't imagining this. He just wasn't.

The waiter came and took their order. 'Is there some kind of irony that I'm ordering the same

things we got for Matt and Marianne?' he asked
as he sampled the beer.

'It's one of the best things on the menu,' she
said simply. 'And I'm getting the other.'

There was a quiet ambience around them.
People at the tables chatted in low voices. There
were no loud boisterous parties and Eli was
grateful.

'What do you normally do on a Friday night?'
he asked her.

She was thoughtful for a few moments. 'Watch
TV, allow my cat to make a fool of me, or read
a book.'

'What about parties, or nightclubs?'

'I did that when I was a bit younger. I'm past
that. I don't mind the occasional wine bar. Or I
went to one of the observatories at night, on a
tour where you can see all the stars and realise
just how small this planet is. I liked that.'

'I did that Night at the Museum thing when
I was younger—when you sleep next to the dinosaur bones in a museum.'

'Oh, wow,' she said enviously. 'That must have
been great.'

'It was. But my friend snored, and another
friend had an accident. Kind of spoiled the
mood.'

She leaned back. 'I would have so loved that.'

'The snoring, or the peeing?' he teased.

'Don't be silly. Just the experience. Lying there, looking up at the dinosaur bones and wondering what life would have been like if we'd lived at the same time as the dinosaurs.'

'Only a mere sixty-five million years in between.'

She took a bite of her salmon. 'You're nit-picking now.' She tilted her head. 'But you're a bit like that, aren't you?'

He put a hand to his chest, feigning mortal offence. 'You wound me. Just because I pay attention to the details doesn't mean I'm a nit-picker.'

She looked up from under her thick lashes. 'That's exactly what it means.'

The conversation flowed easily. The food was delicious, and as two hours slipped away, Eli finally started to find some peace.

As they walked out to the car, he turned to her. 'I guess I need to face the fact that Matt isn't likely to get to work to train a new vet any time soon.'

She held his gaze as she opened the driver's door. 'So where does that leave us?'

Us. That was what she said. And he knew she meant the practice. But it didn't stop a good percentage of his skin from prickling. Would he ever be ready for another *us*?

The roads were quiet. Aurora turned on the radio and selected a channel that played soul music as they made their way back to the vet practice, where her own car was.

Eli contemplated all the things he could do next. None of the options made him happy—at least he didn't think they did.

'I hadn't planned on staying, but if I want the practice to successfully continue, I'd need to stay for at least a year after I recruit a new vet— maybe even longer.'

'You make it sound like a prison sentence,' she said simply.

The words made him cringe. 'I just have mixed-up memories about this place. After my mum died, my dad was juggling things. I know that he loved me but, to be honest, I think he loved the practice more. He missed out on a lot of things that are important to a kid.'

She shot him a glance while she drove. 'Did he have any help?'

'Matt and Marianne. He and Matt shared the workload but—' he shook his head '—it seemed like whenever there was something important for me: a football final, a school concert, a big exam—' Eli sighed '—there just always seemed to be an excuse for him not to be there. Always an emergency, or a planned surgery, or he'd forgotten to put it in the calendar. And the thing is, I know Matt and Marianne reminded him. I know Matt always offered to do whatever the vet thing was at that point.' He closed his eyes tight for a second and scrunched up his face. 'I can even remember a conversation I wasn't supposed to hear, when he asked Matt to swap with him, so he didn't *need* to come.'

'Oh, Eli,' she said softly.

He opened his eyes again and gave another soft shake of his head. 'So, Matt and Marianne would come. I'd stay there if he was called out in the middle of the night. And they were great. I think, in truth, they were as frustrated with him as I was.'

'Do you think you reminded him too much of your mum?'

He turned to look at her, watching how the final remnants of purple light cast a glow across her skin and hair. 'I wondered that at one point, but I don't really resemble Mum at all, I have much more of my dad's features.'

'Maybe you have your mum's mannerisms, or habits. Apparently, I've inherited some of my gran's traits, and even sometimes, when something comes out of my mouth, I cringe, because I can almost hear her voice in my head saying it too.'

'I guess I might have. I just still have a deep-down feeling that I had a dad who loved his work and the animals more than his family.'

'Do you ever wonder if you might get like that?'

He leaned his head against the window. 'Don't miss anything with those punches, Aurora,' he said, a light tone still in his voice.

She shot him a worried glance. 'Sorry, I really should think before I speak.'

'One of your gran's traits?'

She gave him a grateful smile. 'Absolutely.'

They pulled up outside the practice and both climbed out of the car. Eli walked around the bonnet and met her halfway.

Now, she was lit up from the back, streaks of silver, purple and deep navy behind her. She sensed it, and glanced over her shoulder and laughed.

'I guess someone thought we needed good lighting,' she said easily.

They locked gazes, and Eli took a step forward. It seemed entirely natural.

'Thank you,' he said in a low voice. 'For this afternoon, and tonight.'

She stepped forward too. Now, they were only inches apart. She lifted her hand and put it on his arm. 'It's fine. I was glad to be there. I don't think you should have gone alone.'

He focused on the hand on his arm. And all the sensations that were shooting along his nerve-endings. His eyes moved slowly from her hand, up her body and to her face.

Their gazes locked again. Green eyes. Big green eyes with dark lashes. Dark? She must be wearing mascara.

As they stood in silence, Aurora licked her lips. This time she took a mini step forward. Eli's hand lifted and rested on her hip, just as her own palm tightened on his arm, almost as if she was willing him even closer.

They moved in unison, lips brushing for the briefest of seconds before they locked entirely. Her hands wrapped around his neck, the length of her body pressed up against his.

He didn't want this kiss to stop. He refused to let any memories of the last person he'd kissed invade his mind at this moment. He refused to let himself be swayed by the fact Aurora was a workmate.

He was wise enough to recognise the different circumstances. There were no similarities here. He could concentrate on this.

The feel of her lips against his. The pressing of her hands around his neck and back. His lips moved to her face, her ear and her neck and she let out the tiniest groan. He could taste her perfume on his lips, feel it with every inhale.

She let out a breath and stepped back, nervous laughter filling the air between them. Her pupils were dilated, the green of her eyes nearly invisible.

'Whoa,' he said, trying to catch his breath.

'Whoa,' she repeated, a broad smile across her face.

She blinked for a second, obviously letting the cool night air clear her head. 'Not how I expected the evening to end,' she said.

He wasn't sure about her tone. Was it regretful? Was she questioning herself? Did she have doubts about their kiss?

'Me neither,' he said. He couldn't be untruthful. 'But I'm not sorry.'

She licked her lips again, and he wondered if he should invite her in. But Aurora was too quick for him.

'I have a cat to get home to, and you have a puppy to attend to.' She let her shoulders relax, and she swung her bag over her head. 'I'll see you Monday?' she said.

'Sure,' was all he could reply. Was she dying to get away from him?

She gave a wave of her hand as she headed over to her own car. ''Night,' she called as she climbed in and drove away.

''Night,' the reply came on his lips. But he stayed where he was and watched as her car headlights finally faded into the distance.

What on earth would Monday bring now?

CHAPTER SIX

ANNE WAS MANNING the phone with an annoyed look on her face. Aurora was immediately on edge. Did Anne know that she and Eli had kissed the other night?

She immediately stuck her bag in her locker and came through to the main reception. 'Want me to take over?'

Aurora had learned that although all tasks were supposed to be shared, there were some things that Anne just didn't enjoy doing. She had a pad and a calculator and a spreadsheet open on the computer. Aurora recognised the software immediately. Wages? Was there an issue?

The wages software was usually easy. Hours entered. Checked by the accountant, salaries paid.

'I think I made a mistake. Matt should still be getting paid sick leave. Eli is on the pay-roll now, you and I have our hours inputted, but Frankie called to say he hadn't been paid for his final week's notice. He had holidays owed, so he should still have been paid. But I can't find the glitch in the system.'

Aurora nodded. 'That's right, I remember us having that conversation. Do you want to swap? I've got Mrs Pringle coming in to get some information on getting her cat spayed. Do you want to have the chat, and I'll have a look at this?'

'Perfect,' said Anne, out of the chair like a shot.

Aurora smiled. She really didn't mind. She was sure she would figure things out.

Half an hour later, Bert sniffed his way around the corner towards her. 'Hey, little guy,' she said, picking him up and setting him on her lap.

She was still petting him as Eli came around the corner. 'Hey,' he said easily.

'Hey,' she replied, unable to help the smile on her face. She hadn't slept a wink the other night. Too many what-ifs had floated through her mind.

It had been spending the afternoon and evening with him that had just drawn her to Eli, stronger than ever. She'd seen him vulnerable at Matt and Marianne's, the love they all had for each other very apparent. The meal had been delicious, but the conversation in the car?

It had felt as if she was finally getting to know Elijah Ferguson for real. There were some real mixed-up feelings about his dad. She could tell he was doing a lot of unpicking himself. But he'd been honest with her. Now, whilst she might not really understand the resentment he felt deep down, at least she could empathise. Coming back here was tough for him. And the realisation on the same evening that he would likely have to stay here for at least the next year—was that what had done it for her? Knowing this flirtation and attraction might have a chance of lasting more than a few weeks?

It had certainly helped. She'd never been the kind of girl to look for very short-term. She liked a chance to get to know someone and be part of their life on a regular basis.

And the kiss? The kiss had taken her breath away. Literally.

She'd wanted to get in her car and drive away? Absolutely not. Had it been the right thing to do, for him and for her? Absolutely yes.

She'd needed that space. She needed to work out how things would be at work between them. Some people couldn't handle a relationship with a workmate, but she certainly hoped that she and Eli were adult enough to work this through, because she actually wanted to see where it might go.

It honestly felt like something was sparkling inside her. She hadn't really wanted to attempt any kind of real relationship in the last few years, since her assault on set, and the stalking fiasco afterwards. The long-term counselling had given her the rational grounding that she needed. She'd learned to forgive herself, and respect that she wasn't responsible for either incident. She'd learned to apportion blame appropriately. She'd started to trust herself again. She'd been so cautious ever since both incidents—probably to the point that she recognised she pushed people away, and likely hadn't given anyone much of a chance in the last few years. But she was getting there.

And this was the first time she'd *wanted* to give someone a chance. She'd felt the buzz, the connection, that she hadn't felt in years. But this time she was older, more confident, and surer of where she was in life, to take it and grab it with both hands.

But would Eli grab it with her?

'Are you up for going back to the Fletchers' farm today?'

'Of course,' she said as he moved over, closer to her.

'I know you were planning on talking to Matt about it. Did you get a chance?'

His face was serious. 'Yes, he's definitely thinking it could be a risk of TB due to the badgers. He said the farm was due to do their bovine TB testing next month. We need to get up there, find out as much as we can, and see what we can do next.'

'Want me to get changed?'

He nodded then glanced down at the screen. His gaze narrowed. 'What are you doing?'

She was a tiny bit surprised at the edge in his tone. 'Wages, swapped with Anne. She said there was a flaw somewhere, and Frankie hadn't been paid for his last week. I've just checked, amended it, and forwarded it on to the accountant to check.'

He blinked, nodded and said in a low voice, 'Okay, go and get changed and I'll meet you back down here.'

Was that slightly awkward? She wasn't sure, because her head was so full of the potential consequences of finding bovine TB on one of the farms they served. It was massive and would involve a huge team of professionals to work through the issues.

'I've phoned Don Fletcher to let him know that Matt suspected there potentially could be an issue with the water or food supply transferred by badgers. He's devastated at the potential threat to his herd, but happy to do everything he can.'

'We'll need to check the cows, isolate them, contact the authorities and arrange testing.'

He nodded. 'It's going to be a long day. Let's go.'

If she'd expected some lightness today, Aurora knew she wasn't going to get it. A flirtation at work was nothing. This was someone's livelihood and herd. She had to be completely focused on work, and play her part to gather as much information as possible.

It was late evening by the time they got back to the practice. They'd spent hours at the farm, talking to Don, checking the cattle, making sure they were sufficiently isolated. It did look as though the food supply could have been compromised. Some badgers were either ingenious or sneaky, and potentially could have infected the food or water supply. Since there was more than one herd, there had been long discussions about making sure there was no crossover of usage of areas. Plus, ensuring that no cattle, equipment or milk could leave the farm. In amongst all this were the huge array of phone calls to Defra, the government agencies and departments who dealt with potential bovine TB, Public and Environmental Health and the Animal and Plant Health Agency. It was exhausting.

They'd followed all the personal cleansing and disinfection rules on entering and leaving the farm as a precaution, and the testing was arranged for the next day, along with one of the specialist vets. But both of them still felt grubby. Aurora was pulling at her tunic top and jacket.

'Want to grab a shower?' Then he looked at her again. 'How far away is your place? Do you want to just stay here, rather than drive home tonight, since we need to be back at the farm early?'

She hesitated, but only for a second, because it did make sense and she was already feeling too tired to drive.

'Okay, thanks.'

Aurora was familiar with the layout of the rooms. The place had previously been some kind of small family estate, the downstairs mainly converted to house the practice, with upstairs occasionally used by visitors or staff.

She understood Eli had been staying there rather than use the vet's house next door, which he hoped would attract someone to the new job, but she hadn't really seen much of how he was living.

By the time she came out of the shower, she could smell something cooking in the upstairs kitchen. She knew this one was rarely used and, as such, was immaculate, or at least it had been until Eli arrived.

He had white flour on the tip of his nose. Bert was in the corner of the kitchen, drinking from his water bowl then making short work of his food.

'Making pizza,' he said, clearly a bit frazzled.

She changed into new scrubs, which she always kept at the practice. This pair were older and well worn, so more comfortable than usual. 'From scratch? You didn't have anything frozen?'

He gave a shrug. 'I lived in Italy. I know how to make real pizza.'

'You know how to make a mess,' she joked.

He looked around the kitchen and nodded in agreement. 'I certainly do. Let's hope it's worth it.' He opened the fridge and pulled out a bottle of white wine. 'Want some?'

'After today? Abso-blooming-lutely.'

He poured two glasses and kept peering into the oven, checking on the pizzas. After a few more minutes he pulled them out and put them on wooden boards. Instead of sitting at the small table in the kitchen, he gestured with his head. 'Want to go through to the sitting room?'

'Sure.'

The sitting room window was wide open, letting the warm summer evening air filter into the room. Eli set the boards and pizza cutter down on the low table in front of the grey sofa, then flicked on the TV. 'Football, football or football?' he asked in a jokey manner.

Aurora glanced at the clock. 'One of the history or mystery channels, please. I'd like to hear about Machu Picchu, the Pyramids, the Rosslyn Chapel or the Titanic, please.' She gave him a quick wink. 'I'll even watch something about an old shipwreck if you can find it.'

He walked swiftly through to the kitchen, grabbed their wine glasses and sank down beside her. 'Do you know how long I've wanted to hear those words from someone else?'

'I guess I'm just permanently nosey and curious,' she said. 'I'd love to work on one of those shows.'

It was a throwaway comment. And she had considered working in the background of TV, rather than as an actor or presenter. But for a second she froze, wondering if she'd just revealed too much.

But Eli clearly didn't take too much from the comment. 'Me too,' he said with a spark in his eyes. 'Can you imagine how much more doesn't reach the screens? It must be fascinating.'

He grabbed a slice of pizza and took a bite and she did the same.

'Wow,' she said as the flavour hit her tongue. 'That's amazing.' She stared at the pizza base suspiciously. 'It's got a bit of bite to it.'

He nodded. 'The tomato base sauce has a hint

of chilli—more like an Arrabbiata sauce? I think it makes it tastier.'

She nodded in agreement, her brain swirling. This was the time. This was the time to mention her previous job, and why he might think that he recognised her. She could just do it casually, ask him if he'd ever considered a different career before training as a vet. But now she knew the answer to that would be no. It wouldn't be an easy subject to introduce that way.

There was a noise from the corner, and they both turned their heads. Bert had snuggled down in his basket and was comfortably snoring. They started laughing at the same time.

'A snoring puppy?'

'Lucky me,' said Eli. 'I'll sound his chest tomorrow, but I think it's just how he's lying with his little head tucked in.'

He took another breath. 'There's two extra bedrooms across the hall. You can pick whatever one you like to sleep in.' The words came out so quickly that they almost ran together. Was he nervous?

She picked up her wine and took a sip. 'Perfect, thank you. I'm just glad I didn't need to do that drive home. I might have fallen asleep.'

'What about your cat?'

'Miss Trixie will be fine. I already texted my neighbour to feed her and go and check on her.'

'You called your cat Miss Trixie?' There was scepticism in his tone.

'She's a rescue, she came with the name. But I have to say, The Queen would probably suit her better. She thinks the rest of the world is there to do her bidding, and I swear she looks at me with disdain most of the time.'

'The world of cats,' he sighed. 'One day, scientists will be able to understand a cat's thoughts, and I genuinely think we will all be horrified by how badly they think of us all.'

She laughed. 'Oh, I can almost guarantee it.'

He reached out and touched her arm and she flinched. She hadn't even had a chance to have a single thought. It was just slightly unexpected, and it was her body's automatic response.

Eli's face changed instantly. 'Aurora, I'm sorry.'

She reached for the spot on her arm and shook her head. He'd shared so much about himself in the car. Wasn't it at least time she shared a little bit in return?

'It's me,' she said. 'I had an experience when I was younger that came as a shock.'

He was sitting very still on the sofa next to her.

'It makes me nervy. I feel as if I have a spider-sense that tingles sometimes.'

'With me?' he asked, looking horrified.

She gave him a soft smile. 'No, not with you, Eli. But if anyone touches me and I'm not expecting it, my body just reacts.'

He closed his eyes for a second and just breathed. 'I am so sorry,' he said. 'That should never have happened.'

'No,' she said calmly, 'it shouldn't. But sexual assault happens to women all over the world. And I was, like most, shocked at the time, blamed myself, and didn't want to report or complain.'

'So, what happened?'

'I finally admitted things to a much older member of our team, who had much more direct methods. He reported him, and when others heard, other women stepped forward to say he'd grabbed them, or cornered them too.'

She gave a sigh. 'Actually, just knowing that made me feel a whole lot better. It wasn't just me. He'd been the same with other women, and I absolutely wasn't to blame.'

Eli gave a careful nod. She could tell he was treading warily, but she'd noticed he'd stuffed a clenched fist under his leg on the sofa.

'Did he get sacked?'

'Yes, and no reference.'

'Did the police do anything?'

She'd been in South Africa at the time. But police forces the world over weren't much different.

'An alleged sexual assault is difficult to prove. Unless a grab has been particularly forceful it sometimes won't leave a mark. I didn't want to put myself through a trial, where some might have doubted me, or thought that I deserved it.'

'That's awful.'

'It was. But I survived it.'

And a lot more too, she thought.

'I had no idea,' he said earnestly. 'I'm sorry I alarmed you.'

The screen flickered in front of them and the titles for a documentary on the *Marie Celeste* appeared. Aurora felt partly relieved.

'Do you know what I could do with?' she asked.

'What?'

'A hug,' she said simply. 'Refill my wine glass, let me slump on the sofa next to you, watch some interesting TV and not worry too much about what tomorrow will likely bring. I need a few hours of nothingness.'

'I can do that.' He picked up their glasses, walked to the kitchen to refill them, and when he got back to the sofa he relaxed down as Aurora leaned against his side. His arm went easily around her shoulders and she just rested against him.

'Perfect,' she murmured.

* * *

Eli's head was spinning, as his body would quite like to react in a normal way to having a woman he was extremely attracted to this close. But he concentrated hard to try and dampen all his desires.

The documentary passed the hour easily. They sipped their wine, and he enjoyed the heat and feel of her next to him. The curves of her body against his. The clean scent emanating from her hair and body.

As the credits started to roll, she looked up at him with those too green eyes. She didn't even speak, just lifted her mouth to his.

He was tentative. He was wary. Because now he was in new territory. Now, he was conscious of his every move and not wanting to give her any reason to feel nervous. So he let Aurora lead the way entirely.

And she did. As their kisses deepened, and hands brushed against each other's skin, it was Aurora who made the move to swing her leg over and sit astride him, letting him run his hands up her back and touch her smooth skin.

It was Aurora who tilted her head back to give his mouth access to the delicate skin on her neck.

And it was Aurora who positioned herself where she could clearly know the effect she was having on him.

'How about I don't sleep in one of the spare rooms?' she asked.

He tried not to let out a groan. 'You want to steal my bed now too?' he joked.

Her eyebrows lifted. 'I want to steal your bed with you in it,' she replied.

He thought they might take things slow, but she stripped off her clothes on the way to the bedroom and turned to face him as he entered.

'Always so slow?' she teased as she climbed into bed.

Eli had never shed clothes so quickly in his life as he joined her on the bed.

'You sure about this?' He had to ask. He had to make sure they were both on the same page.

'Absolutely,' she replied with a big smile on her face as she pulled him towards her.

CHAPTER SEVEN

TESTING A HERD of nearly one thousand seven hundred would have been a nightmare. But, thankfully, the Fletchers kept their herd segregated, and it was only two hundred cows that could have been exposed.

The seven who were considered symptomatic were tested first, with their tuberculin skin tests to be read in seventy-two hours. In the meantime, Don Fletcher wasn't looking too good himself.

'Don,' said Eli, already knowing what the answer might be, 'do you drink unpasteurised milk on the farm?'

'Every day,' he admitted. 'Public health are sending someone out to test me later today. Me, and Jake, the herd boy. He has breakfast here every morning and we both drink unpasteurised milk.'

'Any symptoms?'

'GP already asked me a few questions days ago. He's ordered a chest X-ray, but the public health person said they will need to look at that and the TB test together to consider a diagnosis. Chest X-ray is booked for tomorrow.'

'What about Jake?'

Don frowned and shook his head. 'Not sure who his doctor is.'

'I'll let the team at public health know and they'll arrange a chest X-ray for him too.'

Don sighed. 'We've reinforced around all the stores and water supply, but it's really too late now. Once bovine TB is in the herd, the cow-to-cow transmission can be high.'

'Let's just wait and see what the tests show.'

Don nodded as Eli finished up all the things he needed to do on the farm that day.

It had been a strange morning. Nice to wake up with Aurora in his arms. Reassuring to notice how comfortable she felt beside him. Unusual to discover how in synch they were in the kitchen in the morning, where both of them had refused to even function before they had coffee.

There had been a serious atmosphere this morning. Because they knew the day ahead was going to be tough. To her credit, as soon as they'd arrived at the farm and after taking one look at Don, who was pale and thin, Aurora had gone with the vet from the Animal and Plant Health Agency, along with one of the farm hands to get things started.

Eli had assisted where he could, then gone back to chat with Don in the farmhouse for a while. Don could already have tuberculosis, which was impacting on his health. But Eli was also conscious of the immense amount of stress and pressure an event like this would cause to a farmer. The health and wellbeing of the farming community was always at the forefront of his mind.

'I'm surprised you're still here,' said Don, in between coughs.

'You are?'

Don nodded. 'I thought you'd cut and run as soon as you could.'

Eli decided to be honest. 'I wanted to, but Matt is sick. I'm not sure if he'll be well enough to come back, and I'm still advertising for another vet. Until all that happens, I have to stay.'

'Do you think you'll get someone?'

Eli raised both hands. 'It's difficult. I might be able to attract someone newly qualified, but even then I'd need to stay and oversee them for at least a year. So, my plans have had to change.'

Don looked at him for a few moments. 'I'm glad to hear that.'

'You are?'

'Of course I am,' he replied. 'If you close, the nearest vet practice is twenty-five miles away. And I don't know those people. Your practice—

Matt's? I've known you both for years. I trust you both. If Matt hadn't been sick, this would all have happened probably some time last week. But I'm grateful that as soon as you both had that conversation you picked up the phone to let me know what you were thinking, and what would happen next.'

'It's what every vet should do.'

'But not all do. I've heard tales from other people that other agencies have just turned up at their farm after the vet has left.'

'I'd never do that to you, Don.'

'I know, son.' He reached out and placed his hand over Eli's. The gesture was small, but meant so much for an old guy like this.

Eli's eyes fixed on their hands. This. This was part of why he was here. He'd never want to let the farming community down. This was part of why he loved his job so much. Working in all parts of the world was great. Learning and get-ting experience with other kinds of animals was also great. But farming was the backbone of so much in Britain.

He'd always known his father had completely loved it. And that, in turn, had made him want to invest his time and energy in different ways, and in different places. But the reality was that he, Elijah Ferguson, loved working on the Scottish farms. And for some reason it seemed as if he was only truly realising that now.

Aurora appeared at the doorway. 'Everything okay?'

Don pulled his hand back and gave her a nod. Aurora walked over to the stove in the kitchen and turned the hob on. 'Barb phoned with strict instructions I was to make sure that you ate, Don. She's left this pot of soup, and said it was big enough for us all.'

Eli moved over to join her, cutting bread from a thick loaf. 'He is looking thin, and pale.' He glanced at Aurora, who was pulling out bowls and had found a soup ladle. 'I'm glad Barb phoned you.'

They exchanged a small smile. He liked how resilient she was, and how she wasn't afraid to jump in and help. One of the farm hands went to round up all the others and plates of lentil and ham soup, along with thick farmhouse bread, were served to all.

'I need to get the recipe for this,' Aurora whispered in Eli's ear. 'I am absolutely rubbish at making soup.'

He smiled in surprise. 'The first thing you're not good at. I learn something every day.'

'The second thing might be pizza,' she freely admitted. 'I've never made pizza from scratch before. Some might say that last night you were just showing off.' There was a glint in her eyes.

'What part?' he immediately joked and laughed as colour seemed to spread up her cheeks. But no one else in the room had noticed. It was as if they were in their own private bubble.

When everyone was done, Eli loaded the dishwasher as Aurora made Don a coffee and cut him a slab of gingerbread that Barb had left.

Something was dancing around in his brain. He liked her. He liked her a lot. But he'd been down this road with a colleague before. Someone who had pulled the wool over his eyes.

Yesterday, he'd noticed that Aurora had been in the practice's accounts. Granted, it was a small place, and everyone might do more than their role. But neither his solicitor nor accountant had mentioned that the wages were done by the staff themselves. Matt had mentioned it. But to Eli, with his naturally suspicious mind, it all seemed a bit strange.

It wasn't as if Aurora had tried to hide it. She'd been upfront and said Anne had been struggling, the last employee hadn't been paid and she was helping. Was it really normal for a vet nurse to do the wages?

Maybe it was because he'd been working in other countries. Most other practices had been much bigger than this one at home, and there had been finance offices to deal with all the wages. He couldn't remember what had happened in the past. He'd been too young to care and then, as a teenager, he'd only been interested in the animals, not the running of the practice. This could be entirely normal.

But he'd need to check.

He hated he felt like that. But he couldn't push it away. It was just too important. If he was going to be around for the best part of a year or more, he really needed to get a better handle on the day-to-day running of the practice. He should have done it before now.

'What's wrong?' Aurora asked.

'Nothing,' he said quickly.

'Are we ready to go then?'

He nodded and they followed all the cleansing and disinfectant rules before they left the farm. As they drove along the road Aurora gazed at the scenery.

'You know, I was thinking. You could make some improvements to the practice.'

'What do you mean?' He wasn't sure why he was instantly alarmed.

'It's just that, last night, I noticed upstairs has clearly been renovated in the last few years. Downstairs, the practice looks a bit tired by comparison.'

'You think?' He hadn't really thought about it

at all. He'd worked in some state-of-the-art practices, and some middle of the road. His father and Matt's practice had never really entered his thoughts at all.

'It's just, as you're advertising and looking for someone new, if you brightened the place up a bit, got some new equipment, it might attract some new candidates.'

Okay, what she said made sense.

'And you've already made a start on the kennels out back.'

He nodded. She was right. The kennels at the back had been used during the good weather to sometimes monitor pets or keep them until their owners returned to collect them. They'd been pristine in years gone by, but had obviously been less of a priority in recent times. It had taken some blood, sweat, tears and some timber to resurrect Bert's playpen, but he could take some time to do the rest, particularly when it was nice weather.

'I could do the rest of the kennels,' he said slowly.

'Then we could think about the two treatment rooms. The doors could do with replacing, and maybe a new sink in one. The floors in both could be replaced and they could do with a coat of paint each too.'

'Are you turning into one of those house

shows on TV, where they throw you out for a couple of days, then the owners come back and find they've turned a library into a disco?'

She gave a small laugh. 'Not quite. I just think it might help things. And I'm happy to help. I can put a few things through the accounts.'

It was like a chill going through his veins. He tried to be rational. But being a victim of a crime, and realising how many tiny tells there had been that he'd missed, had imprinted on his brain.

Last night had been the best night he could remember. Aurora's lips on his, her skin against his, and that feeling of connection that he'd always been seeking but had never found before. All of that was currently skewing his rational thoughts.

Aurora must have noticed the way his hands had tightened on the steering wheel because she gave him a strange look. 'Forget it, don't worry. It was just a suggestion. Why don't you wait another few weeks and see if you get any applicants?'

His heart ached. She was trying to help him. And if this was genuine she might think him ungrateful. But if this was something else— something cold and calculating that he'd missed before—then there was still a chance to stop things.

As he drove along the last mile to the practice his mouth was bone-dry. He couldn't pick up the phone to Matt. It wasn't fair. He couldn't ask him the questions he wanted to ask. Like how well he knew Aurora. If he'd checked her references and qualifications.

Then, cutting clean through those thoughts, was something else. Was this it for him? Was this how he was going to spend the rest of his life? Second-guessing. Never trusting, always questioning what anyone told him.

He wanted to believe not. Maybe it was just timing. Maybe it was just because this was the first time he'd really let someone close since Iona. It could be that he would always have been like this next time around—and Aurora was just caught in the emotional crossfire.

He hated the way that sounded. He hated more the way it felt.

'I'll think about it,' he said, knowing his words might sound a bit abrupt. 'I'm still thinking about a lot of things with Don Fletcher's farm. Let's deal with that first.' He looked sideways. 'And, there's some other things to pick up. Jack Sannox and Rudy for one.'

She turned to face him. 'Do you trust me to do that?' There was an edge to the question.

'Of course I do,' he replied.

'Then I'll go tomorrow if we're not back at the Fletchers' farm all day.'

He licked his lips, trying to be rational and calm. He was a vet. There were a number of crises right now for his clients. Some huge in volume, and some smaller—but with equal emotional value.

'I would really appreciate that,' he said steadily. And he realised he meant it. Jack Sannox and his wellbeing mattered to him. From everything he'd seen of Aurora in her professional capacity, he had absolutely no reason not to trust her. If she was worried about Jack, she would let him know.

Aurora's phone buzzed and she pulled it out of her pocket as they reached the practice. She frowned. 'It's Anne, saying that patient with the diabetic cat is insistent on talking to me again.'

Eli's head shot around. 'Are you worried?'

He watched as she took a deep breath and focused on the practice building instead of him.

'Let's just say that my spider-sense tingles around him.'

'Then we don't see him. I'll ask Anne to tell him that our books are full, and to divert him to another practice.'

He could see the wave of relief wash over her, not just from the visible welcome slump of her body. This had been hard for her—hard for her to admit. If they hadn't connected last night, might she not have told him?

That was the last thing he wanted for staff that worked for him.

'Thank you,' she said, her voice a little shaky.

He reached over and took her hand. 'Any and every time,' he said firmly. They sat for a few minutes while she collected herself, then she gave a big sigh and fixed a smile on her face.

'Let's go back inside.'

They were met by Bert at the door, who looked as if he'd been up to mischief. Anne simply raised her hand from the desk. 'Don't ask,' she said.

Eli smiled and walked over to her. 'The man you texted Aurora about, the one that's been insistent about dealing with her?'

Anne nodded.

'Can you phone him back and say unfortunately our books are full, and refer him on to another vet practice, please?'

Anne met his gaze. She was one of those characters that didn't need things spelled out to her. 'No problem, I'll do it now,' she said, picking up the mobile handset and moving into another room.

'What have we got this afternoon?' asked Eli, as Aurora walked back through to Reception.

'Two dogs. Both are being considered for

breeding. Eye checks done. DNA tests completed with no concerns, but both need to be sedated to get their hip and knee X-rays completed for grading.'

'What kind of dogs?' Eli asked. This was routine work for this practice. Not every practice had the qualifications or skill to do these kinds of tests, but it was something both Matt and his father had insisted on continuing. Mainly because it helped keep up the quality of dogs being bred, and it was profitable.

'One Labrador, and one dachshund,' said Aurora.

He gave a nod. 'No problem. I'm going to spend some time writing up the notes from the Fletchers' farm, then I have a video call with some of the other agencies at five o'clock tonight. Give me a nudge, will you? I might forget.'

'We'll be finished the X-rays long before then, and I'm happy to stay later if either of the dogs takes some time to come out of their sedation.'

'Thank you,' he said, meaning it. She really was an excellent staff member.

Anne came through once he was settled at the computer. 'Anything you want to tell me?' she asked.

Eli felt heat rush into his cheeks. How on earth could Anne already know that something was going on between him and Aurora? His father had always said not to underestimate how astute she was, but that was usually in relation to owners who didn't quite tell the whole story about something.

'Er…' he started, stuttering over his words. 'I might have started dating someone,' he said.

It was like being a fourteen-year-old again. Anne had just started at the practice then, and used to leave him tongue-tied. But he was a fully grown adult now. Should he really tell her this stuff? She didn't have any right to know.

She'd just blindsided him.

A smile appeared around her lips. 'Anyone I know?'

He took a breath. 'Maybe,' was his response as he straightened himself up and got ready to explain that this really wasn't something to discuss.

But Anne rested a hand on his shoulder, the smile disappearing from her face. 'I was talking about Matt,' she said sadly. 'Marianne said you visited last night.'

His face fell, and he inwardly cringed. Of course she'd meant Matt.

'But I welcome the other news,' said Anne, in a way that only she could.

He moved his hand and put it on hers, looking up. 'He wasn't great, Anne. Much sicker than I realised. His colour was almost translucent, and he's lost so much weight he hardly looks like

Matt any more.' He sighed and looked down for a second, before he had a moment of realisation. 'But you knew that, didn't you?'

She gave a slow nod. 'I would never have said anything to you, until I knew you'd been to visit.' She paused for a moment, her face the most serious he'd ever seen it. 'You have to think carefully about the future, about what makes you happy, Elijah.'

'I know,' he admitted. 'And I still don't know what that is.' He put his hand on his chest. 'I still don't know if I have the heart to be here.'

Anne stayed silent for a few moments. 'Only you can answer that question.'

'I know,' he sighed. 'But there's so much going on right now, and so much to think about.'

'You're right. There is. But at some point you have to take some time to stop and think. Just promise me that.'

He gave a nod and Anne slipped her hand from his and disappeared back through to one of the treatment rooms.

Aurora was feeling odd about things. One part of her was fizzing with excitement. She'd only ever experienced telling one potential partner in the past about her sexual assault. The reaction had been confused, with a real reluctance to try and reach out to her. She got that. It scared some people. But Eli's reaction last night had been different.

He'd accepted what she'd said. He'd been angry—even though he hadn't said anything. He'd been sorry she'd had that experience but had been supportive. Then he'd still reacted to her touch. With caution, maybe. But his touch had been just what she'd needed.

It had revitalised her. It made her feel real again. Parts of herself that she'd kept hidden had been unleashed. She'd also felt good about revealing a part of her history with Eli. He'd taken it well, and she knew she still had to tell him about her past career.

She was just worried that he would think less of her. The reactions of colleagues at university and in placements had made her so glad that she'd worked as an actress under another name. Even those colleagues who'd said they admired the TV show had still treated her as a bit less. It was actually shocking how the world seemed to assume that anyone who was an actor wasn't clever. She hated that.

She could already tell that Eli was beginning to trust her professional judgement and competence. She didn't want that to be compromised.

Then there was the stalking. It was another horrible dark hole in her mind, and if she really wanted to have a relationship with someone it would have to be revealed.

She didn't want to think about any of that right now. She wanted to live in the moment. Let the electricity continue to spark between them. See where things led. For a few moments today she'd wondered if something was off. But then again, when was the last time she'd been in a relationship? Maybe she was just rusty. Maybe she should make more of an effort?

They worked closely together the rest of the afternoon. Both dogs were sedated and X-rayed without any concerns. The little dachshund took a bit longer to recover completely and Aurora was happy to stay with him until he was wide awake and his owner came to pick him up.

Once she handed him over, she walked back through to one of the offices, where Eli was still working on the computer.

'Ready to finish?' she asked.

He looked up. 'Nearly—why, is something wrong?'

She shook her head. 'I just wondered if you want to do something.'

He must have got a hint she had something planned. 'Like what?'

'Well,' she said slowly, not trying to hide her smile, 'I know it's summer. But there are two options. We could head to Portobello Beach for chips and ice cream, or we could head into the city and catch one of the last tours of the graveyards and the dungeons. It should be dark enough by then.'

He leaned back in his chair and folded his arms. 'Wow. Two great suggestions.' He looked out of the window. 'What time is the last tour?'

'About eleven,' she said, 'and they last about an hour. We could grab dinner some place first.'

He closed his eyes for a second. 'Or we could take Bert with us and go for a walk on the beach. It's years since I've been to Portobello Beach,' he said with a smile.

'How long?' she queried.

'Maybe eighteen or nineteen years. I wonder how much the place has changed.'

'Chips and ice cream it is, then?'

He nodded. He seemed genuinely happy. 'Let me go and get changed. Do you want to get changed too?'

She nodded but said, 'My house is on the way. Can we stop there and I'll run in and grab some clothes, and check on Miss Trixie?'

'No probs,' he said. 'Give me fifteen minutes. I'll finish this, jump in the shower and grab Bert.'

Bert could clearly sense something was going on as he started to get excited. Aurora wrestled him into his harness for the car journey, and Eli appeared a few minutes later in jeans, a white T-shirt and brown leather jacket.

All it did was remind her just how handsome he was. He looked like something from an aftershave ad.

This time the car that Eli pulled from his dad's garage was an old-style silver Aston Martin.

'You have to be joking,' she said.

He shook his head. 'Perfect for a wee drive to the beach.' He laid a blanket over the back seat and secured Bert in place. 'Let's go.'

She had to give him directions to her house. It was slightly odd for her. After her stalking experience, she'd been careful about what name she used, and how many people actually knew where she lived. She'd kept it to a minimum. She directed Eli through her village and to her cottage. She loved her home, was proud of it. Her garden was immaculate. And although the house had new windows and shutters, it had a traditional wooden red front door.

'Your place is lovely,' said Eli as he pulled into the driveway.

'Thank you,' she replied with a smile. 'Do you want to come in while I get changed?'

He gave a nod, then glanced at Bert and changed his mind. 'I'll just take Bert for a walk around the garden first.'

Aurora nodded and got out of the car, leaving

her front door open behind her and dropping her bag on the table near the entranceway. She ran up the stairs, took the quickest shower in history and grabbed some clean clothes out of her bedroom, while Miss Trixie watched her with apparent indifference from the top of the bed.

The temperature was still warm, so she grabbed a pair of white capri pants, flat shoes and a white-and-green-striped T-shirt. As she went back along the corridor she noticed Bert and Eli still outside. Her eyes caught sight of a pile of mail from the day before that she hadn't even looked at. But the thing that caught her attention was her stage name—Star Kingfisher—on one of the envelopes. Not only that, it was addressed to her stage name, with the actual house address. It hadn't come via her agent like most mail did.

Her skin chilled. Had someone tracked her down? She swallowed hard. Her stalker had gone to jail but had been released less than a year later. She hadn't heard anything from him in years. Could he have tracked her down again?

She felt sick.

'Ready?' came Eli's voice from outside.

She stuffed the letters into her bag. She'd look at them later. Eli was outside, as Bert sniffed around the garden.

'Didn't you come in?' she asked.

'We got as far as the sitting room,' he said. 'Like your purple sofa, by the way. But Bert was sniffing around too much. I was too scared he'd relieve himself on your nice purple rug.'

She smiled, because she couldn't quite laugh yet.

He held up one hand as she stepped outside. He hesitated a second then gave a little shrug of his shoulders. 'Just wondered if you wanted to bring anything for tomorrow.'

Now, her smile broadened. 'Are you asking me to stay overnight?' she teased.

'Only if you want to.'

She stood for a few moments, letting him think she was considering things, before turning and going back in, putting tomorrow's food out for Miss Trixie. She grabbed another few things, flung them in another bag then went back out to lock her door.

As she turned around, something about the car flashed through her head. 'Has that car been in a film?'

Eli gave a bashful smile. 'One nearly the same was in one of the James Bond films. I'm not sure how or where my father ever got an Aston Martin from, but he only took it out on special occasions.'

'So, is that what I am,' she asked as she climbed in, 'a special occasion?'

He laughed as he started the car. 'Of course.'

The drive down to Portobello Beach was beautiful. The sand was a dark yellow and the tide was currently coming in with blue waves and white peaks as they found somewhere to park.

'Will the car be okay here?' asked Aurora, feeling a little worried.

'It's a car,' said Eli easily. 'And—' he spun around, holding his hands out '—the people here are good. They're not going to make off with a James Bond car. Remember what happens to any villain that tries.'

She frowned for a moment, trying to remember what did happen to people in those films, but her mind was a blank. And she was secretly pleased that he liked her home, even though he hadn't got to see much of it.

They moved along the street, which was filled with locals and holidaymakers. She could hear an array of different accents and even though it was late in the evening there were still some children down on the beach, playing on the sand.

Eli lifted Bert up into his arms. 'Right, little guy, let's see what you make of the sand, and the sea.'

They made their way down onto the beach. As the tide was part way in, they didn't have to walk too far. Bert loved it. There was no other way to describe it. He looked at the sand between his paws for a few moments then had a dig, sending sand flying. Next, he rolled in it. Then, when they moved closer to the sea, he didn't hesitate to run straight into the waves.

'He loves it!' declared Aurora as he splashed her again and again. She took off her flat shoes and walked through the waves with him, grabbing the lead from Eli. 'This is freezing though,' she yelled over her shoulder as Eli crossed his arms and stood laughing at them both.

A crowd of twenty-somethings walked past, with one nudging the other and then all turning to look at them. Were they looking at him? Or her? Nope, they were definitely looking at Aurora, with her dark red hair flying madly about and her laughter as she interacted with Bert.

'Your feet will take an hour to heat up,' he said, shaking his head as they both made their way back to him.

'They won't. These shoes, they're actually made from a kind of recycled material. They can be washed and are waterproof.' She gave him a wink. 'What's more, I have them in twenty different styles and colours.'

He groaned. 'I knew there had to be a flaw somewhere beneath that perfect smile.'

She moved closer, cutting out the wind between them that was blowing briskly. 'You think I've got a perfect smile?' she said.

She was trying to pretend to be cool, but the man in front of her was one of the most handsome guys she'd ever seen. A few other women had glanced in their direction. With his blue eyes, scruffy styled hair and designer stubble, he was attracting lots of admiring looks. She almost wanted to make sure everyone knew he was with her.

He put his arms at either side of her hips as she moved closer. 'I think your smile is pretty great,' he said. Her hair, which was whipping around her face, was caught by him, with a strand tucked behind one of her ears. 'And I think the colour of your hair is stunning.'

'You do?' They were chest to chest now. She decided it was time to tease him again. 'So, last time you were at Portobello Beach, did you kiss a girl?'

He threw back his head and laughed. 'I wish. But I'm doing it this time,' he added, before putting his lips on hers.

And for the first time in a long time Aurora thought she might get a chance at happy ever after.

CHAPTER EIGHT

THE FIRST LETTER seemed almost like a mistake. A fan apologising for sending a letter to her address, which was more of a query to ask if Star Kingfisher would be returning to the vet series. The second letter asked why she was living her life under another name, and if she was trying to keep her identity a secret.

Aurora tried to phone the police officer who'd dealt with her stalking case—but he'd moved on, and no one else could really help.

She was left jittery and unnerved.

In the meantime, work was getting busier by the day. Bovine tuberculosis had been confirmed in some of the Fletchers' herd, which sent a huge chain reaction of next steps. All the other cattle were tested, with no milk or beef allowed to be sold or moved from the farm.

The impact on Don Fletcher's farm was huge, along with the repercussions for his workers. He himself had been diagnosed with TB, as had his younger farmhand. The system was designed to recompense farms affected by bovine TB. However, all things took time.

In the meantime, all the surrounding farms had concerns, and testing was arranged for them too. Aurora and Eli spent huge amounts of time on virtual meetings, coordinating with all the agencies involved.

Eli himself was clearly stretched. He was doing the work of two vets. There had been contact from a French vet who was interested in coming to Scotland, and there had been a few enquiries by those due to qualify. Two had arranged to come and see the practice, but Aurora was already convinced that working alongside one vet wouldn't appeal to a new graduate. They usually wanted to find their feet in larger practices with bigger support networks.

With all this happening around them, it seemed as if there wouldn't be any time for Aurora and Eli. But, strangely, this wasn't quite true.

There was a consistent and ongoing connection between them. When a pet had required overnight care after surgery, Aurora had volunteered to stay over. It happened on rare occasions, when animals had a slower recovery from their anaesthetic, or their owner wasn't quite equipped to take care of them.

Eli had waved his hand. 'I can do it. I'm here anyway.'

'But you have a million other things on, and you need to get some sleep,' she'd insisted. 'I can set the alarm and get up a few times in the night to check. It's fine.'

And she did. Of course, she hadn't minded at all that they'd decided to take the little cat upstairs and held it on her lap as they watched TV on the sofa, his arm around her shoulders and her head on his neck.

It was such a comfort. She was just trying to get her head around the fact she could actually have something real. Seven years ago, she'd been the apple of a number of guys' eyes—but it was hard to separate who was interested in her, Aurora, as opposed to who was interested in tabloid fodder and headlines about the latest popular actress.

She didn't have to worry about that with Eli. He only knew her.

The next week passed easily. They continued to work together, supporting the members of the farming community around them, learning how to create a new team. Anne watched with the permanent hint of a smile on her face. She said very little about it, but occasionally remarked on how the practice was beginning to run smoothly again.

They were making plans to head into Edinburgh for the evening when the doors of the practice burst open and a teenage girl ran in, clutching something in her arms.

'I can't believe it. I am so sorry. I never even saw him.'

Aurora and Eli were on their feet in seconds, Aurora wrapping her arm around the girl's shoulders as Eli eased the little animal from her arms.

It was a dog—a puppy, and almost a carbon copy of Bert. One of its legs was clearly broken and the only sound it made was whimpers.

Aurora steered the girl to a chair. 'Tell me what happened.'

'It just ran in front of me.' She crumpled and put her hands on her face. 'I hit it with my car. I've only had my licence for six months. I didn't have time to stop.'

'Where on the road were you?' she asked gently. She was trying to be patient, but knew she had to assist Eli urgently.

The girl explained. It was near the spot that Aurora had climbed through the woods to find Bert.

'Phone your mum or dad,' she said. 'Ask them to come and get you, and let us take care of the puppy.'

She hated to do it, but she had to leave the girl in the waiting room to go and look after the puppy. She dialled Anne on her mobile as she took the few steps into the treatment room. It was likely they would be busy for the next few hours and the practice would be left uncovered. Anne answered immediately, and said she would be there in ten minutes.

Eli's head was bent over the puppy as she entered the room, washing her hands and grabbing a trolley with IV supplies.

He spoke gently. 'He's so scrawny,' he said, then pressed his lips together.

Her heart ached. 'She knocked him down near where I picked up Bert. Do you think they could be from the same litter?'

'Highly likely. Can't imagine how this one has managed to keep going.'

The little dog's ribs were clearly visible. Eli had his stethoscope out and was listening to the puppy's abdomen. 'Sounds okay.' His eyes flickered to the back leg. 'It's badly broken.'

She knew what he was going to say. The little puppy was so scrawny and thin; he had to contemplate if it could withstand an anaesthetic.

They worked together, shaving the hair on one of his front legs, inserting an IV to give fluids for the puppy's too fast heart rate and low blood pressure. Aurora put some oxygen on, and drew up some pain relief for Eli to insert.

'What do you think?'

The little guy's whimpers started to die down. Eli took the opportunity to draw some blood and handed it to Aurora. She knew automatically what to check for. This was another way to ensure the puppy would be fit for anaesthetic.

The practice had been able to screen their own bloods for a number of years and it saved time on the more regular tests. Complicated blood tests still needed to be sent to more specialised labs, but in times like this the ability to check for themselves was crucial.

'He's a little bit dehydrated,' Aurora said, showing him the blood results.

He nodded. 'I'd like to weigh him,' said Eli. 'I need to know how much anaesthetic he could tolerate. This could be touch and go.'

'Let's give the opioids another minute to kick in,' said Aurora. 'I'll need to lift him onto the scales.'

Eli was gently stroking the little dog's back. 'There, there,' he said. He met her gaze. 'Operating might not be a good idea. There's a chance he won't tolerate the anaesthetic. And we already know he doesn't have an owner. Not when he looks like this.'

Aurora gave a nod, but pulled the scanner from the nearby drawer to check for a microchip. Of course, there was none.

Eli looked her steadily in the eye. 'We'd need

to look after this guy ourselves in the rehab period before we hand him over to a rescue centre.'

'We can do that,' she said steadily. 'I think we have to give him a chance.' Their gazes remained locked. 'Why have one Bert, when we can have two?' she said with a smile.

Eli had been upfront to begin with about not wanting to stay. But since their visit together to Matt's, it was as if all parameters had changed. They both knew he'd have to stay for at least a year. Recruitment was still open. Another vet had yet to materialise.

Before that visit, he'd asked her to consider adopting Bert. But nothing had been mentioned since. Maybe she was jumping to a whole host of conclusions here. Maybe the fact they were in a relationship was clouding her judgement. But she didn't think so. He'd revealed part of himself to her. She understood why he struggled with the memories of his past here. And he, in turn, had been a good personal support about her assault. It gave her faith that she could continue to move past that and form a meaningful relationship.

There was a noise as the front door opened and Anne bustled in. She was her usual reliable self, her eyes catching sight of the young girl in the waiting room and their own situation in the treatment room.

She gave them a wave of her hand. 'Go and do what you need to do,' she said.

They disappeared into the theatre. The little dog was anaesthetised, his leg area prepped and draped, with the theatre lights adjusted to give Eli the best possible view.

Before cutting the skin, he took an X-ray to see what he was dealing with.

'It's broken in two separate places. I'll need to plate and pin.'

Aurora knew that would take a few hours. They worked together steadily, her assisting where required and monitoring the little dog's breathing and vital signs. There were a few scary moments, when the little dog had a burst of tachycardia during the procedure. But things settled down.

Eli kept a close eye on the puppy's blood pressure, ensuring adequate IV fluids were given, since he was already a little dehydrated. 'Thank goodness there's not much blood loss. I'm not sure his body could take it.'

He leaned back, arching himself to stretch out his spine. As he finished his delicate work he looked at Aurora. 'Do you think there's any chance there are more of them?'

'Don't say that.' She shuddered. 'It's bad enough I missed one. I'd hate it if there were others.' She licked her lips under her mask. 'Do you think we should go and check later?'

He paused for a second, then looked down again. 'Let's wait and see how this little guy does first. We need to get him through this before we worry about anything else.'

After a while, Anne stuck her head through the door. 'The young girl was picked up by her mum and dad. I've to give them a call to let them know how the puppy is.'

As Aurora gave her a nod, Anne paused for a second. Even from the other side of the theatre, Aurora could see the flash of concern in her eyes. 'There's another query about the wages that I can't answer.'

Aurora didn't hesitate. 'That's fine, leave it for me. I'll sort it later.'

Eli gave her a fleeting gaze, and for the briefest of seconds she thought she saw something strange in his eyes. But, next second, the alarm sounded and they both turned their attention back to the puppy.

'We should give this guy a name. We can't keep calling him dog, or puppy.'

'Why don't you pick the name, since I picked Bert?'

'You picked Bert because you said it was someone good that you worked with?'

She nodded.

'Okay, in that case, this guy can be Hank.'

Aurora couldn't help but smile. 'Hank?'

'Yes, when I worked in Maine, I worked with a vet called Hank. He was one of the good ones. Great accent. Great values. I really admired him.'

Aurora looked down and stroked the little one's head. 'Okay, Hank. Here's hoping you can wake up soon and we can introduce you to your brother, Bert.'

Finally, the surgery was finished and the wound stitched. Anne came into the room. 'I'd made scones at home, so just brought some when you phoned. I knew you'd be here a while. Go and have something to eat and I'll monitor him while he recovers.'

'Hank,' said Aurora. 'We've called him Hank, and think he could be Bert's brother. The accident was in the same kind of area.'

'Oh, dear,' said Anne, stroking his head. 'He does have the same distinctive white flash on his head.' She gave a little nod. 'Off you two go.'

They walked back through to the kitchen, where the plate of scones sat, along with the kettle boiling. Eli pulled off his cap and sighed as he sat down. 'We'll just need to wait and see how things go.'

Aurora went to sit down, then changed her mind. She walked through to the back kennels and shouted Bert in, picking him up and cuddling him while she sat at the table.

'You okay?' Eli asked, pouring the tea.

'Yeah,' she sighed. 'Just wishing that the day I found Bert, I found Hank too, and all of this never happened. That little guy has been foraging for himself for nearly a month. It doesn't bear thinking about.'

Eli carried the tea over and reached across, rubbing Bert's head. 'You can't think like that. At least you found Bert. He's doing great, aren't you, guy?'

Bert lifted his head into the air and sniffed. 'Is that the scones you smell, or is it your brother?' asked Aurora, giving him another cuddle.

Eli split the scones and spread them with butter and jam, putting them on two plates, and she continued to hug Bert.

'What will we do with Hank over the next few days?'

'I can ask Anne to do some extra hours. I'm sure she'll be happy to.'

'Okay then.'

'Because…' he met her gaze with a smile '…we will need some time off.'

'We will? What for?' she asked with a smile, warmth flooding through her like a comfort blanket.

'I've booked us onto something.'

'That sounds mysterious.'

'There's a graveyard tour in Edinburgh, by bus. Does the underground stuff too. But also some drinks and snacks as we do the tour. Thought we might give it a try.'

'That sounds like fun. You thinking about the Scottish weather again?'

He gave a shrug. 'You know what it's like. The graveyard and vault tour are probably best in October and November. This seemed like a fun added extra, and it doesn't leave until eleven at night.'

'Why do I have a feeling there's something you're not telling me?'

He gave a wide grin. 'It might be billed as a horror comedy tour.'

She laughed. 'Is the horror the actual comedy?'

'I guess we'll find out.'

'When are we going?'

He pulled a face. 'I'd booked for two nights' time. That was before Hank though. I'll check with Anne, to see if she can cover or not. If not, we can change it.'

Aurora nodded and, as she ate her scone, lifted the pile of notes that Anne had written this afternoon while manning the desk and answering the phone. Most were for repeat prescriptions. Anne had already printed them, and was just waiting for Eli to sign. She and Aurora would dispense and phone the owners back to let them know to collect the medications. There was another with some follow-up details Aurora had asked about a dog's diet. One query about a sick parrot. And a final one that made her stop cold.

Caller on the answering machine asking to speak to Star Kingfisher? Quite insistent. Must be wrong number.

A chill swept over her entire body. *No, not here too.*

She closed her eyes for a second and tried not to throw up. Could this be her stalker again? The kidnap attempt hadn't been a physical kidnap attempt, but the police had got wind of it, and foiled it. There was clear evidence of the stalking. Aurora had texts to her phone—even though she'd changed her number a few times. Letters sent to her house. And emails to her agent, and to her own private email account. All of them bombarding her to continue in her role, when it had been announced she was leaving the series.

She hadn't actually had to appear in court with her stalker. She'd been protected from that. And she'd never seen him in person. Just his police mugshot, and a picture of him entering court seven years ago. Would she even recognise him if she saw him now?

That actually scared her more than she wanted to admit.

She had to tell Eli. She had to tell Anne. It made her insides curl. Not only would she be letting them know she'd had a past career she'd kept from them, but now she was potentially bringing trouble to their door. What on earth would they think of her?

'Aurora? You okay?'

She opened her eyes and took a quick gulp of tea to soothe her bone-dry mouth.

She tried to be rational. Matt knew about her past career. When she'd applied for the job—although she hadn't written it on her submitted CV—she did tell him what she'd done in her late teenage years. He'd brushed it off easily, asked a few questions about the animals she'd interacted with on set, and what she'd learned about them. But once she'd answered his questions she'd said she was just trying to have a new life, and he'd said he respected that, and wouldn't mention it again.

So she hadn't been totally dishonest.

She took a deep breath. 'Yeah, there was just something I was going to mention—'

But she got cut off. Anne appeared in the doorway. 'Eli, I need you.'

They were both on their feet in an instant. Animals could crash after anaesthesia. The most common signs were tachycardia, low blood pressure—both of which had been borderline for Hank—and hypothermia, which he was exhibiting now. Anne had wrapped a silver blanket around him.

'I'll give something else to reverse the anaesthetic again. Can you increase the rate on his IV fluids please, Anne?' asked Eli, checking the wound, then taking out his stethoscope to listen to Hank's chest again. They were all silent for a moment, before he pulled the stethoscope from his ears. 'No fluid in his lungs. No heart murmur, just a consistent tachycardia.' He touched Hank's head tenderly. 'Just a little guy who might not have the pull to get through the other side of surgery. Maybe we shouldn't have done it. Maybe this was cruel?'

It was the first time she'd ever heard Eli doubt anything he'd done as a vet. No practitioner was infallible. There were always times they had to weigh the odds and hope they worked in their favour. Had she pushed him to do this?

She put her hand over his. 'This wasn't cruel. This was us doing our best and trying to give Hank a chance.'

Anne gave a slow nod. 'There's the human side too. If I had to tell that teenage girl that we'd had to put the puppy down, I doubt she'd get over it. Hank had a chance, and he still does.'

Eli gave a slow nod and sighed. 'I just hate these parts of the job. He's just so scrawny. I've used minuscule amounts of drugs on him, as I have to be so careful about what his body can tolerate.'

'I have an idea,' said Aurora. 'Give me a minute.'

She ran through to the kitchen and picked Bert out of his basket, holding him firmly in her hands as she walked back through to the recovery area.

Bert made a little noise, as if he picked up the scent as soon as he came in the room. He started to scrabble a bit, but Aurora held him firm. 'No, honey. Hold still, let me take you over to him.'

Hank murmured too, coming around a little more from the anaesthetic now the drugs were kicking in, and sniffing the air.

Eli and Anne smiled as Aurora brought Bert nearer, talking quietly in his ear the whole time. She held Bert close enough to rub his head next to Hank's. Bert desperately wanted to get closer, but she didn't want him to knock Hank's leg, so she manoeuvred around, allowing them to see each other, to lick each other's face, and to touch with their paws.

'It's probably a million times better than any drug,' said Eli, giving her a smile that warmed her heart.

It struck her just how much she wanted this to work. She'd never met anyone like him before. And although she needed to tell him about her alternate identity, she was still glad that he just knew *her*. And liked her.

What had started out as rocky had blossomed very quickly into something special. And as she watched him lean over Hank, stroke his head and talk to him, she realised she loved this man. She actually loved him.

His too long, scruffy hair that she could run her fingers through. The stubble on his face that would scrape her cheek. The feel of his muscles flexing under the palm of her hand. That look from those blue eyes that made her insides want to melt.

She could do this. She could stay here. She loved this place already, but had never really considered it for ever. But now? With Eli? It could be.

But could she be his for ever too?

Trust for her had been so hard since her past experiences. But trust with Eli had always seemed unquestionable—even when she hadn't liked him those first few hours, she'd never felt unsafe. She'd never been worried.

But there still seemed to be an edge to Eli. Something that lay deep down beneath the surface. She wondered sometimes if she really knew everything about him.

But then, he didn't know everything about her.

That would have to change.

But as she watched him take care of Hank, while still holding Bert close to her chest, she knew there was a time and place for everything. And this wasn't it.

CHAPTER NINE

'I THINK I might fall asleep,' said Eli, as they climbed onto the decorated bus.

'Me too,' Aurora whispered as they were led to a table on the bus where a skeleton was in one of the seats.

'Guess this guy won't mind,' joked Eli, as he slid in next to the skeleton and slung an arm around its shoulders.

'Maybe that's what we all look like when we get off the bus,' joked Aurora, as one of the attendants approached with a tray of cocktails, all smoking and bubbling.

Eli picked something green and Aurora something peach-coloured and they both took a sip. 'Ouch,' laughed Eli, his cheeks drawing together. 'Well, that one is a bit strong.'

Aurora's eyes started to water. 'Mine too.' She gave a little choke. 'One of these will definitely be enough.

The last few nights had been tiring. Hank hadn't settled well. They had no idea where he'd been sleeping in the woods, or how long Bert and he had been separated from their mother, but he was difficult to get to sleep.

Both of them wished Bert could be in beside him. But Bert still had jumpy puppy traits that meant he could unwittingly hurt his brother, so they were waiting until he'd healed a bit better. They'd also spent a whole afternoon tramping around the woods to ensure there were no further puppies abandoned, but had found nothing. It had been a relief.

As the other passengers loaded and the guide gave an overview of what would happen, Eli studied Aurora.

He didn't mean to. He just did it every opportunity that he got.

She was beautiful, with her skin slightly tanned and a few freckles across her nose, her dark red hair and bright green eyes, he actually couldn't believe he'd got this lucky.

More than that, she had a good heart. She was feisty. She didn't put up with any nonsense. She had a real understanding of the farming community that actually put him to shame.

He'd underestimated her in the first few seconds of meeting her—but he'd never been that foolish again since.

Every day he spent around her, he learned more about himself, and more about her. Part of him felt as if coming here had been cathartic. Part of him felt as if seeing Matt had been a wakeup call, to be grateful for life, and all that was in it.

But meeting Aurora had been the icing on the cake.

He'd never experienced a spark like this. He'd thought he had. But now, with hindsight, he realised he'd been fooled. Every time he looked at her, he had a fresh wave of emotion. She affected every part of him. His senses seemed to go into overdrive around her. Just one whiff of her perfume was enough to send goosebumps across his skin and blood rushing to other parts of his body.

It was time to talk. Time to feel his way to seeing if he could make this more permanent. He still had questions. He still had trust issues. He wasn't sure they would ever go away. But those were his issues, not hers.

Aurora hadn't given him reason not to trust her.

He wondered if things had just moved too quickly between them. How he felt certainly had. He loved her. He was sure of it. He wanted to work next to her every day. He wanted to take her for a drive in every car in his father's garage. He wanted to replace some of the photographs in the hallway with some newer ones—one of them together, one of them with their dogs. But how would she feel about that?

The bus pulled out. The journey would take a few hours, with some pitstops along the way. They'd go on a visit to Greyfriars Kirkyard and walk to the statue of Greyfriars Bobby. They'd pass Holyrood Palace and go along Grassmarket and close to Edinburgh Castle. They'd go back down the Royal Mile, learning ghastly and ghostly history wherever they went, and finally finish with a visit to the underground vaults.

He leaned back into his skeleton friend as they listened to the comedian. The mood on the bus was light, jovial and the drinks seemed to be going down well.

He took a breath. 'About the practice,' he said.

'Yes?' She looked up straight away.

'You've probably guessed this because you were with me when we visited Matt and Marianne, but I'm going to stay.'

'For good?' There was an edge of hope in her voice. And he cringed inside. His answer should be yes, but he still couldn't honestly say that.

He swallowed. 'I'm going to stay for at least a year, then take it from there.'

'A year?' Was that disappointment in her voice?

'At least. One of the potential applicants looks like a good candidate. You met her—Cheryl

Wood? She, her husband and children are keen to move here. Her husband's a school teacher and they know there are plenty of jobs in the area. She's had some maternity leave during her studies, so qualifies in September.'

'The school term here starts in August. Won't that be too late for her husband?'

'He can work on the teaching bank. Apparently, there are lots of hours, and it will give him a chance to get to know the area, and where he might want to work permanently.'

'Only a year?'

He blinked and put his hand on his chest. 'I'm still not completely sure if I want to take over Dad's practice. Working here has been better than I thought. I'll always be known as David Ferguson's son, but I'm beginning to feel as if I can put my own stamp on the place.'

'Does that mean you'll let me decorate?' She'd already shown him some plans and given him some costs to update parts of the practice.

'I showed them to Matt, and he likes the idea.'

'You did?'

'I did.'

'But you still can only say you'll stay for a year?' Her voice had softened slightly.

'Aurora,' he said softly, 'I don't want to make false promises. I think this could work out. I think I might like to stay. But, until I know for sure, I only want to promise that I'll stay for the next year.'

She looked at him steadily and he continued.

'You have to know that a big part of why I want to stay is you.'

She sucked in a breath. 'Me?'

He gave her a smile. 'Absolutely.'

The bus jolted and both their drinks slid across the table, Eli barely catching them with one arm.

She let out a laugh, then leaned forward, her face serious as she reached out and touched his hand with her fingers. 'I'm glad you want to stay because of me, but you have to want to stay because of you too.'

'And that's the part that's getting there. You just have to give me a little more time. There are a few other complicating factors that mean I can't take over the practice completely. I have to let Matt and Marianne look after my dad's share for now.'

'But Matt's…' She let her voice tail off and pressed her lips together.

His other hand met hers. 'And I'll cross that bridge if I need to. For now, I don't.' He took another breath. 'And if I do decide I don't want to stay, I'll talk to you about it first.'

Her brow creased. 'So you can say goodbye?'

'No, so I can ask you if you want to come with me.'

She stayed very still. 'That sounds serious.'

'I am serious.'

'We've only known each other for a short time.'

He gave her a level look. 'I know that, but I know how I feel.' His insides were doing somersaults. It struck him that having this conversation on a bus, where both of them were essentially trapped for the next few hours, meant things potentially could go horribly wrong.

'How do you feel?' she asked, her fingers clenching under his.

He kept his voice steady. 'I feel like I've met someone that I can picture myself spending a lot of time with.'

Her voice was equally steady. It was almost as if she was challenging him. 'Spending a lot of time with, as in a fling? Or spending a lot of time with, as in something else?'

The question was close to the bone.

He didn't hesitate. 'Definitely something else.'

A slow smile started to spread across her face, and she leaned over and rescued her peach cocktail. 'Is that something we should drink to?'

'I think it is,' he said, picking up his green cocktail and clinking it against hers.

The two of them were smiling, and Eli had to untangle himself from the skeleton to lean across the table and put a kiss on her lips. Her lips were cold and sweet from the cocktail, and he instantly wished there wasn't a table between them.

'When can we get off this bus?' he groaned.

Her eyes gleamed as she pulled her lips from his. 'I have to see Greyfriars Bobby. I have to do the unthinkable thing of touching his nose.'

'I don't think we're allowed to,' he whispered. The act of touching Greyfriars Bobby's nose by visitors was frowned upon, and had caused the paint to have to be restored on numerous occasions.

'You can distract everyone else,' she said.

He shook his head in mock horror. 'I'm a Scotsman. I don't think I can do that. It goes against the grain.'

She rolled her eyes and signalled to the waiter on board for another drink. 'It's just your luck—' he grinned as the waiter plonked a blue glass down in front of her, again with smoke pouring from it —to end up with a patriotic Scotsman.'

She raised her eyebrows at him in disdain, then looked warily at the cocktail. 'I have no idea how they do this, but I like it. Okay, if you're going to fail me at Greyfriars Bobby, then we need to talk about our dogs.'

It was that little word. *Our.* It struck him straight in the gut and he liked it more than any other word on the planet.

'What about our dogs?'

'They're brothers. I don't think we should separate them. They've been through enough trauma.'

'Ah.' He lifted his own glass, which was looking remarkably empty. 'You're going to play the trauma card, are you?'

She smiled. 'To be honest, I don't think I need to, do I?'

He shook his head and smiled. 'What kind of vet would I be if I didn't have a rescue dog?'

'And what kind of vet nurse would I be if I didn't encourage you to have two?'

He raised his glass to her anyway. 'To Hank and Bert?'

She clinked his glass and lifted the still smoking blue liquid to her lips. 'To our boys.'

CHAPTER TEN

THEY COULDN'T HAVE timed things better. Aurora had called the pet hydrotherapy pool this morning and there was a cancellation. Things were quiet today, so they'd left Anne at the practice with Bert, and she and Eli had brought Hank to the treatment centre.

Hank was improving slowly. His wound had healed perfectly but he was walking with a slight limp. Eli had X-rayed him again to check the position of the plate and it was perfect. But a visit by a pet physio had told them that his back leg muscles were imbalanced and needed building up and the best way to do that was in a pool with hydrotherapy.

Since their colleague knew they were professionals, she'd agreed to set the programme and teach them how to assist Hank, with only a few check-in sessions with herself. The one thing she had been clear about was that the first time they immersed the little guy in water they both went in with him.

Neither of them had objected to this, and Aurora had changed quickly into her red one-piece swimsuit and tied her hair up in a pony-tail, before emerging and meeting Eli, in his dark swimming shorts, at the door.

'Shouldn't we be in Ibiza, dressed like this?' he joked.

'If only,' she sighed. 'But then I would need a shedload of sunscreen, so I can live with this.'

Hank was sniffing the air, obviously smelling the chlorine.

'Does this count as a date?' She smiled as she took her first few steps into the small pool.

The treatment centre was perfectly equipped. There was a small pool that could be used for any pet that needed immersion or swimming therapy. Then there were smaller set-ups with treadmills underwater to allow the dogs to exercise without the full weight on their legs.

'This would have to be one of the weirdest dates in history,' said Eli as he stepped into the water, let his shoulders go under and then held out his arms for Hank.

He whispered in his ear as he took Hank from her. 'Check out the beginners. All the others have wetsuits on.'

Aurora looked around and pulled a face, realising they were the only people with actual swimsuits on. 'Well, we're new to this. And, let's face it, we'll do anything to help our boy build up his muscles. If I have to come here every week and put on my swimsuit, I will.'

Hank's front legs were paddling in the water. He seemed to be a natural.

'Hey,' she said, 'did I ever tell you about my red Lab, Max?'

"You mentioned him."

She raised her eyebrows. 'Well, one day, Max and I went for a walk around the boating pond back home. I took him regularly along a river walk and he would bound in and out of the edges of the water, actually skipping, but he'd never really swum. Then one day we walked around the boating pond, and I swear he took a look and then just soared.' She made a motion with her arm. 'He actually soared through the air and landed straight in the middle of the boating pond.'

Eli looked at her. 'I take it he swam?'

'Oh, no.' Aurora shook her head. 'He sank like a stone.'

'But all Labradors can swim.'

'No one told Max that.'

Eli started to laugh. 'What did you do?'

'What do you think I did? I jumped in to save him. Pulled him up, and my boy, he hadn't jumped in at the edge of the boating pond where there were reeds and sand. No, he'd jumped in at the end where there was a concrete wall. I had to push him up over it, then try and haul myself up.'

Eli started to laugh. 'That must have been fun.'

She gave him a hard stare. 'I was like a giant squid. It's safe to say it was not the most elegant moment of my life.'

Eli couldn't stop laughing and Hank looked up in surprise. 'Don't worry, little guy,' he said. 'You look like you can definitely swim.'

They both watched Hank, who seemed to like the water and didn't seem fazed by it at all. Aurora gave him a kiss on the head. 'Who's a good boy then?'

They stayed in the pool for another ten minutes, making sure Hank was fine, before moving over to one of the standalone set-ups that had an underwater treadmill. One of the treatment centre staff came over and set things up for them, following the plan that had been laid out to strengthen Hank's muscles and improve his range of movement.

Once the tank was full, the treadmill started gently and he walked along with a bewildered expression on his face, licking the dog peanut butter at the front of the tank that was there to keep him focused.

'We'll never get out of here.' Eli smiled. 'If

peanut butter is the standard treat, he'll never want to leave.'

'As long as his leg gets better, that's fine,' said Aurora. She was looking around at all the facilities available. 'I've never been in this place before. It's such a great set-up.'

Eli nodded in agreement. 'I've referred clients to similar places before, but I'm glad we've had the chance to come along and try this out for ourselves.'

They spent the next half hour in the treatment centre, then took turns getting changed, dried Hank off, then moved outside to the attached coffee shop.

Hank was happy to lie at their feet while they sipped their coffee.

'Matt's looking a bit better,' said Aurora. 'He had some more colour yesterday when I dropped off some things for Marianne.'

'He messaged me,' said Eli. 'Said he felt as though the treatment might actually help him rather than kill him now.'

'Chemo is just horrid,' said Aurora. 'I've a few friends that have gone through it. Things are always better when they come out the other side.'

'He has another few rounds still to go.'

'I know. Is there anything else we can do to help them?'

Eli looked at her. He took a breath and reached

out and took her hand. 'And that's what I love about you.'

She blinked. 'What?'

'That you think about other people. And you genuinely mean it. You thought about them right from the beginning, to get Marianne's shopping, and both of them dinner.'

Aurora gave a little shrug. 'Don't think I don't know about you helping them set up new smoke alarms the other day.'

He shrugged too. 'But you know how big a part they played in my life when I was a boy. You've only worked at the practice for the last eighteen months.'

She gave a smile. 'But that doesn't matter. When you meet people—inherently good people—you just know it. And the length of time you know them doesn't come into it. What's important is that you know if you needed help they would give it. And it's why you're happy to step up and do things for them.' She gave a smile. 'Anne bakes for them every week. I don't have that skill set, so I'm happy to do other things.'

Her mind flashed back to first meeting Matt. She smiled. 'You know, when I came for my interview, they were both in the middle of an emergency surgery. I offered to scrub in and help.'

'You did?' Eli's eyes widened. 'Matt never told me that.'

Her brain was currently spinning. He'd used the word *love* a few moments ago, and her heart rate had instantly started racing. A few nights ago, he'd told her he'd stay at least a year, and would ask her to go with him if he left. All the barriers that had been in place in her head were now simply falling away.

Was Eli Ferguson going to be the guy she could take a chance on, and hope for a happy ever after?

Her brain flashed to the interview with Matt afterwards, when she'd told him about her past career, and he hadn't been judgemental at all. He'd actually just wanted to know about the animals and her experience. Maybe Eli would be exactly the same.

She opened her mouth to tell him just as Hank decided to wake up and nudge her leg.

'Oh—' Eli smiled '—that's the toilet training nudge. We'd better go outside.'

She nodded and smiled too. It could wait. It wasn't urgent. It had waited this long after all.

And as they strode out into the Scottish sunshine he slipped his hand into hers and a warm glow flowed through her. Perfect—everything was just perfect.

CHAPTER ELEVEN

IT WAS BUSY. He had to go to Don Fletcher's farm today, as some of the cattle were going to be destroyed and he knew that Don was upset. Public health had also decided to screen the other farm workers who weren't currently displaying any symptoms as a precautionary measure, and Don was upset about that too, thinking he'd put his workers at risk.

Eli checked on Bert and Hank. Bert was running up and down the run, and Hank was nestled in some bedding, catching a little sun. Hank was healing slowly, but well. He was eating and drinking and gradually gaining a bit of weight—his muscles a little stronger every day.

He waved to Aurora, who was on the phone to someone, to let her know he was going, and grabbed the mail on the way out. Matt had warned him the practice insurance was due to be renewed and he wanted to keep on top of it.

As he reached the farm his four-by-four slid a little on a slight build-up of mud. It was a typical Scottish summer with occasional flashes of monsoon type rain. As his car drew to a halt, the mail landed in the footwell.

He groaned and leaned over to pick it up, noticing for the first time that one of the letters was in fact a credit card statement. He frowned, not remembering using the credit card, and tore it open. The total amount made him stop. Four thousand pounds? What? He scanned quickly, not really recognising the names of any of the places where money had been spent.

His mind jammed with a million thoughts— all of them panicking, none of them good. He glanced at the farm, knowing he had a job to do.

This would have to wait.

No matter how much he didn't want it to.

Aurora hadn't gone to the farm today. She was catching up on filing some notes and going through the plans for the updates, making sure she had ordered everything she needed. Two of the deliveries were arriving today and she wanted to make sure she was here to receive them—living out in the middle of nowhere meant having a failed delivery was always an issue.

The practice officially had shorter hours today, with the afternoon off for staff training. But Anne had gone out to see Jack Sannox and

Rudy this afternoon, and Aurora was still keeping an eye on Hank.

The front door jangled, meaning someone had opened it. Her delivery? Maybe. She walked through to find the owner of Arthur standing in the hallway.

'I'm sorry. We don't have any appointments this afternoon. Is something wrong with Arthur?' She looked around him, expecting to see his partner walking up the steps behind him. But they were empty.

And so was the practice. She was alone right now, with the exception of Hank and Bert, and a small rabbit in the back who was recovering from surgery.

Her spider-sense didn't tingle, it yelled.

The man gave her a strange smile. 'Yes, I just need you to go over some of the principles of diabetes again. We're struggling with Arthur.'

'Didn't our vet say we were oversubscribed right now? Didn't you manage to find another vet?'

She was trying her best not to panic.

'We couldn't find another vet locally. Our cat is sick. He needs treatment. He's very lethargic.'

Now, that could be truthful and could happen with newly diagnosed animals.

She gave a small smile, a good vet nurse wouldn't turn a sick pet away. 'I thought you said your gran was diabetic, and you understood things?'

Was that cheeky? Maybe.

'I understand the injections, but that's about all.' There was something about his facial expression, as if it was fixed in place and he was playing a part.

'Would you like to make an appointment to come back and see the vet?'

'He isn't here?' It was a pleasant enough question, but it made Aurora feel as if a million caterpillars were currently trampling over her skin.

'He's out back,' she said automatically.

'I didn't see his car.' The man kept smiling. What was his name again—Fraser?

'He has a lot of cars. His father was a collector.'

There was a long silence as the man kept looking at Aurora. His eyes swept up and down her body, making her feel even more uncomfortable, then fixed on her face.

'I can give you some reading material about diabetes in cats. It's probably best you start there.'

She moved to the computer at the reception desk, searched in the files and started printing things off.

'I think I'd prefer a chat,' he said smoothly. 'I have lots of questions.'

Aurora might not have been in any bad movies, but she'd seen her fair share. This was like one of those, where the creepy guy cornered the heroine.

This was not happening to her. She'd taken self-defence classes a number of years ago, on the recommendation of the policewoman in charge of her stalking case. But right now, all those moves seemed to have vanished from her brain.

'I'll start,' he said easily. He moved his hand and clamped it on top of hers, which was on the reception desk. 'Like, why did you change your name?'

Every cell in her body screamed. Her instincts were telling her to pull her hand away and get out of there. But she actually froze. It was as if something icy chilled her entire body and stopped her from moving.

'I mean, Aurora is nice too. But it's not like Star. And what about the TV series? Nothing has been good since you left. The ratings have tanked. You have to go back. I've even thought up a whole scenario for your character, Tara, so she can get back in the thick of things. And don't you think it's time Tara was the main character, instead of a supporting one?'

Her mouth was dry. She could barely speak.

'I want you to leave,' she said. The words came out strangely. Not like her voice at all.

'That's not very friendly.' He didn't even blink an eye.

Everything she'd hoped for. Everything she'd thought she could finally have. And he was here. Spoiling it.

'Your name isn't Fraser, is it?'

He smiled, pleased to have some recognition. 'Anyone can change their name after a few years. I like Fraser. I think it suits me.'

'You are supposed to stay away from me. There's a restraining order against you.'

He shrugged. 'Different country, different laws.'

'I'm done asking, now I'm telling you to leave.' Her voice had got just as icy as her body felt. But she was angry. She was angry at him for invading her private life and ruining her chance of happiness. She'd run away from this guy once. Now she'd have to run away again. Leave the job that she loved. The home that she was happy in. And the man that she'd told herself it was safe to love now.

He looked around. 'But Star, we've finally got a chance to chat. Let's take it.' He went to move around behind the reception desk, and she reached out and grabbed what was nearest. That was the thing about working in a vet practice—

constant cleaning—and the nearest thing was a mop and bucket.

She swung around with the wet mop and directly hit him in the face with it, grabbing the length of the broom like a weapon across her chest and pushing him square in the chest. He was already staggering backwards, caught off-guard by her movement, as Eli came rushing through the door.

'What the…?' he said as he took one look at the situation and put a foot on the guy's chest to keep him on the floor.

She'd never been so glad to see him.

'Eli, this is Brandon Rivers. He was convicted of stalking me a number of years ago and has decided to come and pay me a visit, even though there is a restraining order against him.'

Eli looked down at the floor. He squinted. 'I thought this guy's name was Fraser.'

'Apparently he's changed it.'

'You didn't recognise him?'

'We never came face to face in the past. And I was protected from seeing him in court. This is the first time we've met in the flesh.'

Eli reached down and grabbed the guy by the scruff of the neck. 'Call the police,' he said.

Brandon turned his head and started yelling at Aurora. 'But Star, you've got to come back to the *Into the Wild* series! They need you. We need you. Tara needs to be reunited with Owen!'

Eli looked completely bewildered as Aurora called the police. She explained the situation in a few short sentences, and they promised to send someone immediately.

Eli had taken Brandon into another room and closed the door, so he couldn't see or shout at Aurora. She had no idea what was being said in there. But even though Eli was here, she still didn't feel safe with Brandon in the same building as her.

Had he followed her home some time? Was that how he knew her address?

It was all so overwhelming, but she was determined not to crumple. Not to sink into the corner like she really wanted to and cry her heart out.

The beautiful life that she'd made for herself was over.

Eli's head was on a perpetual spin cycle. He'd been mad driving back to the vet practice. Mad about the amount of money put on the practice credit cards, which he wasn't entirely sure had been discussed and agreed.

For all he knew, she could have added a million personal things into the purchases and he wouldn't be unable to unpick it. This wasn't how a successful business was run, and he knew that better than anyone.

But when he'd walked in the door to see Aurora fighting off some man, all thoughts had gone out of the window. His instinct to keep her safe had gone into overdrive. Now, he was stuck in a room with a man who didn't seem rational or reasonable, who kept calling Aurora by another name, and she said she already had a restraining order against him. Was this the man who had sexually assaulted her?

It was all he could do to keep his hands to himself. Brandon had made a few shouts about wrongful imprisonment, but Eli couldn't care less. He'd attacked a member of the practice, apparently had history for it, and the police had been phoned.

They could sort it out, and take this piece of trash with them when they did.

He desperately wanted to go into the other room to check Aurora was okay. But that wouldn't be wise right now. He could tell from the look on her face that she wanted to be as far away as possible from Brandon or Fraser, or whatever this guy's name was. Who changed their name?

There was a sharp knock at the door, and a uniformed officer walked in, assessing the situation. 'We can take this from here, sir,' he said to

Eli. 'My colleague outside would like to speak to you.'

The rest of the afternoon passed in a daze. There were conversations about Scottish and English law. A large purple bruise had started to appear on Aurora's hand. She'd been looked after by a female police officer, who'd been sympathetic and ruthlessly efficient. Both he and Aurora had been asked to go to the police station the next day to make formal statements, but for now Brandon Rivers was taken away in the back of a police van.

Eli ran his fingers through his hair as he walked back through to the practice kitchen, where Aurora was sitting, a cup of tea—which looked cold—between her hands.

'Want to tell me what just happened in here?' he asked.

She sat very quietly for a moment.

'Do you at least want to tell me what your real name is?'

He could see the hurt in her eyes. But he had to know the truth. The woman he loved hadn't been truthful with him. In more ways than one. He just couldn't believe he was in a situation like this again.

'My real name,' she said, her jaw tight, 'is Aurora Hendricks.' She was glaring at him now. 'My acting name was Star Kingfisher. I was in a show about vets, ironically. It was called *Into the Wild* and filmed in South Africa.'

As she said the words his mouth fell open. Pieces of the jigsaw puzzle were falling into place. He didn't watch many TV dramas but he had seen snippets of the show—mainly to see them dealing with lions, tigers and giraffes.

'That's why you looked familiar,' he said, not quite believing this.

She kept talking. 'It was the show I was sexually assaulted on, by one of the grips. I left shortly after, but as soon as I came back to England I started to be stalked. It happened over the course of a few months. The police became involved as they uncovered a kidnapping plot, and Brandon Rivers was arrested, convicted and jailed. Part of his bail conditions were that he knew I had a restraining order against him. In the meantime, I wanted a new career. I retrained as a vet nurse and haven't looked back. At least not until today.'

Her voice was quite flat. It was almost as if she was scared to let any emotion out because she was trying to hold things together.

'Are you okay?' he ventured. He had to ask— no matter what else was going on in his head— because it was the right thing to do.

'I don't think I'll ever be okay again,' she said simply. 'I thought I'd put all this behind me. I thought I could forget about it all. But it seems like I'm never going to shake him off.'

Eli sat very still. He had questions. He had multiple questions. Most of all he felt betrayed by the fact she hadn't trusted him enough to tell him who she was. This was the woman he loved. This was the woman he'd planned to spend the next year with—and maybe even more. But after his previous experience, trust was everything to him. How could he even imagine a life for them without it?

'Why didn't you tell me who you were?'

'What did it matter?' she shot back angrily.

'Because trust matters to me. A lot.' He left it there and she sighed, running her hand through her hair.

'You don't get it. At university, some people recognised me from the outset. They treated me as if I was stupid, not clever enough to pass the exams, and they certainly didn't take me seriously. As time went on, I managed to shake off Star—partly because I went back to my natural hair colour. I found out that if someone realised later I'd been on the 'vet TV show' as everyone called it, their opinion of me seemed to fall. It's a thing about being an actress. For reasons that are totally invalid, people seem to think an actress can't be serious about having another career.'

Eli let his head hang down as he tried to take

all this in. He understood that Aurora had been targeted and attacked today. That had to be terrifying. What he wanted to do was give her a big hug and tell her that everything would be okay. But for reasons he couldn't quite explain, the vibe between them had changed.

He took a breath. 'Can I ask you something else?'

'What?'

'The accounts. The credit cards. I got a bill today I wasn't expecting.'

She screwed up her face. 'Wh…what?' It was as if the question had totally thrown her.

'It's thousands. I wasn't sure what had happened.'

She shook her head. 'What's happened is the plans you looked at, and agreed to—the plans that I billed out for you, I've ordered all the supplies. The paint. The new sink. The plumbing. The worktops. The facing. The supplies. It all arrives in the next few days then we can sit down and plan where to start.' Her voice had become quieter as she continued. 'Or at least I thought we would.'

Eli blinked. 'I looked at the plans. I showed them to Matt and told you he liked them. But I hadn't okayed them yet.'

'You had.' She was clearly annoyed now.

He shook his head. 'I wanted his overall approval before starting the work. Then my plan was to get into the details specifically. It wasn't a signal to go ahead.'

The furrow in her brow increased. 'But it was. I have receipts for everything I've ordered. The lists were detailed already. I haven't gone away from them.'

'But you used the practice credit card without talking to me first.' He was trying not to sound angry. He was trying to keep it locked down inside.

'But I thought you'd said yes. I thought you'd know.'

He took a long slow breath as he watched the last part of the life he'd thought he was getting finally crumble around him.

'My last practice went bankrupt. It went bankrupt because the practice manager—who I was dating—ran up tens of thousands of debt, and also took out loans against the practice. I had no idea she was doing it. And I found out too late to save the practice.'

There. He'd said the words out loud.

'But… I haven't done anything like that,' Aurora said. 'I've ordered supplies to update the practice. There's no loan.'

He closed his eyes. So much was whirling around inside his head. He wanted to find the right words. But for now, he actually didn't know what they were.

'This is why trust is essential to me, Aurora.'

She stared back at him. 'What I left out was minor. A small part of my past. I told you about the sexual assault.'

'You think someone being jailed for stalking you is minor?' he asked incredulously.

'No, of course I don't!' she shouted back. 'But you can't judge me, you can't judge us, on your past relationship. A relationship that *you* kept hidden. I'm not her—whoever she is.' She took a breath, and then added, 'And having a practice that went bankrupt? That's a big deal, Eli. That's something you should have been honest about. You know the arrangements here are simple. Anne or I do the wages, send things to the accountant. If you'd said there had been issues in the past, and you wanted to oversee that stuff yourself, we would have understood. At the very least, I could have copied you into every email that was sent so you had a record.' Her voice was shaking, along with her whole body. 'It seems we've both not managed to be entirely truthful with each other.'

There was silence. They both stared at each other, then Aurora stood, the chair scraping on the floor behind her.

'I can't stay anyway. Now that he's found me.

I'll never have peace. I can't be here any more. I have to start over.' Her voice still trembled. 'I thought I'd found something here. Something that gave me a chance of a whole new world.'

He couldn't help but speak too. 'I thought I'd found something too. But trust is the most important thing to me, Aurora. I'll always wonder if there's something else you haven't told me. I don't want to doubt you. I don't want to doubt this relationship. But when you've been in the position that I have, this makes things almost impossible.'

He should stop her. He should try and convince her to stay. But right now, he just couldn't. His brain was still telling him to stop and think. He had to take time to discover how he felt about all this. If he could ever trust her again.

She reached the door and stopped, her hand on the doorframe. 'I'm sorry, Eli,' she said.

He looked at her. 'I'm sorry too.'

It was true. He was. For this. For her. For them. And for this whole situation that neither of them had asked for, or wanted.

And then he let her walk away.

CHAPTER TWELVE

AURORA STARED AROUND her house. She loved this place. She'd made her mark on it. Decorated with plain staples with lots of splashes of colour. She loved her garden. The neighbours. Even the drive to work.

And now? Because Brandon Rivers had this address she would never feel safe again.

But that wasn't the thing that was making her sick to her stomach. Not at all.

It had been the expression on Eli Ferguson's face when he'd been asking her questions. He hadn't cared about her past life as an actress. That hadn't made him think any less of her at all—her fears had been completely unfounded.

But the simple fact that she hadn't told him had been her undoing.

She'd always known there were more layers to Eli. She'd thought—a bit like herself—they had time to strip them back, bit by bit, at a pace they'd both be comfortable with.

She hadn't expected everything to come crashing down around them.

But then the money questions. She'd spent last night tossing and turning, trying to remember the exact conversations. She'd honestly thought the conversation on the bus had been the signal to go forward. But the more and more she took things apart, she realised that she might have got things wrong.

She was horrified when Eli had revealed what had happened to him in the past. But she was even more hurt by the fact he had obviously considered that it might be happening again.

Aurora had always been meticulous about money. It was why she'd been able to buy herself a house outright, when some of her previous co-stars had spent thousands on designer clothes and pricey wines.

The very fact he might have thought… It just made her cry even harder.

She tried to be reasonable. She tried to remember that he felt as though she'd broken his trust. And then he'd found a credit card bill, with items he felt he hadn't authorised.

She'd blown it. She'd blown everything. The best thing she could do right now was get her house on the market and try and find another job.

And while it was easy to consider the job, and

acknowledge the mistake she might have made there, what wasn't easy was the ache in her heart. Eli Ferguson's face would appear in her head for a long, long time. She loved him. She hadn't told him but she did. He was the first man in a long time she'd had faith in, and she'd thought he would keep her heart safe. She'd even started to imagine a future together, no matter where that might be.

She brushed the tears from her face and stood up, looking around her house and realising she would have to get it ready to start viewings.

It didn't matter how painful it was. It was time to move on.

It had been a long night. Matt had been rushed into hospital with sepsis due to an infection in his central line, and Marianne had made a call to Eli.

But things had turned during the night. He'd started to respond to the antibiotics, and his heart rate and breathing had settled back down. Eli had taken Marianne home, made her tea and toast and sent her to bed. It was easy to see exactly how much of a strain this was all putting on her.

He went back to the hospital to check on Matt again and was pleased when the consultant arrived at the same time as he did. The consultant stayed for a while, talking about the fact that the central line had been the route of the infection, and suggesting its removal and another method of delivering the chemo. He'd clearly got the impression that Eli was Matt's son, and neither of them stopped to correct him.

Once he left, Eli sat down and took Matt's hand.

'You should know,' said Matt, 'that I named you as my other next of kin. In case it all got a bit much for Marianne.'

Eli squeezed his hand. 'I'm honoured to be named as your next of kin, and I promise to keep an eye on Marianne.'

Matt leaned back against his pillows. 'You look terrible.'

Eli laughed. 'Thanks. Someone kept me up all night.'

But Matt shook his head. 'It's not that. What is it?'

Eli sighed. There was no point in lying, and if he didn't tell Matt the truth he would then just worry about what might be wrong. So, as succinctly as possible, he told him the truth.

Matt gave him a soft smile. 'It's just a mix-up. A misunderstanding. You're adults. You can talk about that. And hurry up and give the place a facelift. Just be glad Marianne wasn't in charge, she would likely have spent five times as much.'

Eli opened his mouth to object but Matt held up one hand. 'I get to do the talking today.' His face was serious. 'Tell me honestly—how have you felt about being back at the practice?'

Eli took a few seconds to answer. He put his hand on his heart. 'I've enjoyed it in a way I never thought I was capable of.'

Matt smiled, and that meant more to Eli than anything. 'And what's helped you enjoy it?'

Eli threw up his hands and sat back in his chair. There was no point in answering. They both knew the answer.

'Then you have to fight for it.'

Eli shook his head. 'I can't. She wants to leave. She needs to move to get away from this guy.'

'Then find a reason to make her stay. Get a lawyer. I'll give you my friend's number. He's a criminal lawyer and he'll be able to help her. Find a way to keep the woman you love safe, Eli. Because there's nothing else so important.'

His skin prickled. 'I never told you I love her.'

'You didn't have to. I could see it.'

Matt took his hand again. 'Don't make your life just about work, Eli. That's how you'll end up. There's more of your father in you than you like to think. Reach out and fight for the person you love.' He smiled wryly. 'I don't even have to tell you this. You already know. Aurora is a gorgeous girl. Full of fire. Just what you need.'

He lay back against the pillows, clearly pleased with himself.

He waved a hand. 'Now, hurry up. And be sure to tell Marianne I told you off. She likes to be good cop; I'm supposed to be bad.'

Eli stood up and smiled, kissing Matt on the side of the face. 'You'll never be bad cop,' he said.

CHAPTER THIRTEEN

HIS HEART SANK like a stone when he saw the estate agent board in the garden. She'd been serious. She was leaving.

He sat outside the cottage for a few moments, telling himself to stop planning everything. He'd spent all of the drive over thinking of all the ways he could say he was sorry, and ask her to stay.

He had the number for Matt's solicitor and had stopped to pick up a few other things before he'd got here. But he wasn't sure that any of them would work.

She opened the door on the second knock, and he blinked. Her normally immaculate hair was tousled and she had her pyjamas on.

She sighed. 'What do you want, Eli?'

'To talk to you.'

'I'm not sure there's anything left to say.'

'Can I come in?'

'Are you a viewer? Are you offering to buy my cottage?' Her words were sharp.

She licked her lips and paused for a second,

so he took a chance and pointed to the car. 'And can I bring our boys in?'

Her bottom lip quivered. 'Hurry up,' she said, before turning and walking back inside.

He collected Hank and Bert from the car, putting them on their leashes, but carrying Hank instead of letting him walk.

When he went inside the house and closed the door, he could see Aurora through the patio doors that led out to the sheltered garden. Toilet training was still a work in progress for the puppies and she knew that. He walked through towards her, and she held out her hands for Hank. He nestled in her lap while she patted him and looked him over.

'I've missed you,' she whispered to him, as Eli let Bert off the leash to run around the garden while he settled in the chair next to her.

'I've missed you,' he said.

She looked at him. He handed her the phone number. 'Matt asked me to give you the name of his friend, a criminal lawyer who will help you.'

She reached out and took the paper. He could actually sense a little relief from her. 'Thank Matt for me.'

He nodded. 'He also told me off.'

'He did?'

'Said our argument was a misunderstanding. And he's right.'

'The money part?'

He nodded.

'I've gone over and over that in my head. I honestly thought you'd told me to go ahead.' She shook her head. 'But that's not the part that bothers me. It's the fact you thought I could be like your ex.'

He winced because he knew she was entirely right. He put his hands up. 'You're right, and the truth is I know you're nothing like my ex. But the experience jaded me so much that I had trouble seeing past it. I was duped. And I have felt such a fool ever since. For the last year I've had trouble with any new friendship because I always wonder if someone's aim is to con me.'

Aurora looked at him with pity. 'That's no way to live a life. You were unlucky.'

He looked her in the eye. 'But me being unlucky affects the life I can lead for the next few years. I can't take over the practice, I can't be a partner. I can only be an employee.'

'And why's that bad?'

'It's not. But being bankrupt is a stain that will hang over my head for years. I won't be able to get a mortgage in the next few years.'

'I don't need a mortgage. I own this place outright,' she said easily.

'I'm just trying to be honest with you,' he admitted as Bert came up and nuzzled at his knee.

'Not only am I a crap boyfriend, I'm also not a very good catch.'

There was the hint of a smile around her lips. 'You're not the only one who let the past affect them.'

His gaze met hers. She took a deep breath. 'I hated that when I told vet colleagues in the past about being an actress—or even if they found out on their own—they just seemed to think less of me. I hated that. I was serious about my job, and didn't want every question about when I was going back to South Africa.' She shook her head. 'Then there was the other stuff. I guess I was trying to forget all about it, to distance myself from it. It was reported in the press at the time, but two weeks later it was all forgotten about.'

She leaned her head on her hand. 'Except by me.' She looked truly sad. 'When the police told me about the kidnap threat I was terrified. You have no idea the thoughts that went through my brain.' She gave him a sad smile and shrugged. 'I'm an actress. I have a vivid imagination.'

'I can't imagine,' he said, a wave of sympathy flooding over him. She must have been terrified. How on earth could he even understand that?

'So when he appeared again...' She swallowed, and he could sense she was struggling. 'I felt like a fool—because I'd never seen him in person, and then he'd already been in the practice, and was that deliberate or am I just the unluckiest person in the world that he turned up where I was working?' A tear slid down her cheek, and he reached over and took her hand.

'If you hadn't appeared…' She shook her head. 'I don't know what I would have done.'

'Aurora Hendricks, you were doing a *spectacular* job,' he said. 'You were like some kind of kung fu fighter. I don't think the guy knew what had hit him.'

'It was pure adrenaline,' she admitted. 'I vomited later, and slept for hours.'

'Well, I'm glad I did appear. You don't deserve that. No one should treat you like that. You deserve, and are entitled, to feel safe.'

She sagged a bit further into her chair. 'But where does that leave me?'

'It leaves you with a sorry excuse of a boyfriend who made a mess of things, but loves you very much and wants you to stay.'

Her bottom lip started to tremble again.

'I will do anything I can to keep you safe.'

'But you don't want to stay,' she said in a cracking voice.

'What I want is to be where you want to be,' he said without a moment's hesitation. He leaned towards her. 'I started to love this place again,' he admitted. 'But a big part of that was you. If you want to stay then I want to stay. If you want to start afresh somewhere else then I'm happy to do that with you.'

'But you would be leaving behind your father's practice.'

'And I'd find a way to make my peace with that. My priority is you.' There was a nip at his ankle and he bent down and picked up Bert, who licked his cheek.

'I am the man who was so shameless that he brought our children with him to help him plead his case. That's how desperate I was.'

Aurora looked down to where Hank was still on her lap. She kept stroking him. 'If I honestly can't feel safe once I've spoken to the lawyer, you'd be willing to move somewhere else with me?'

'Absolutely. I love you, Aurora. Your happiness is what counts.'

'What about our boys?'

'If we need to get them passports, we can.'

She smiled. 'I love you too. And if can, I want to stay. I love working here. I love the community. I love the job.'

He moved in front of her, kneeling and resting his forehead against hers. 'It's you, me and our boys against the world. How does that feel?'

'That feels like for ever,' she said as her lips brushed against his, and he kissed her and didn't let go.

EPILOGUE

THE GUESTS LET out gasps of surprise and gave a round of applause as Hank and Bert trotted proudly down the aisle towards the groom. If dogs could smile, they were currently smiling.

'I can't believe you trust your dogs better than me with those rings,' Eli's childhood friend and best man whispered in his ear.

Eli kept his gaze on his dogs as he spoke out of the corner of his mouth. 'You lost your front door keys seven times in school. How many times have you had to replace your driving licence? And tell me right now where your car keys are.'

John looked momentarily panicked then shrugged his shoulders as he gave a casual smile. 'Oh, go on then, trust the dogs.'

Eli bent down to pat each of his beloved dogs on the head as they arrived at the top of the aisle, each with a bow around their neck, with a ring attached.

They looked very pleased with themselves, and sat eagerly at Eli's feet, waiting for treats.

The music changed and Eli stood up, watching as his bride emerged at the bottom of the aisle. Her dark red hair was pinned at the sides but cascaded down her shoulders. He took a breath, trying to remember to keep going as Aurora moved down the aisle towards him, her father beaming proudly.

Her dress was stunning. Cream, and off the shoulder—Bardot-style was what she'd told him—with a fitted waist and stunning satin figure-hugging skirt. Although she wore a veil, it didn't cover her face, but instead framed it, letting him know just how lucky he was.

But he already knew that.

Their wedding was a little unconventional. All pets had been invited to the outside ceremony. The Scottish weather was behaving today and blessing the guests with some bright sunshine. Jack Sannox was there with his new rescue dog that Aurora and Eli had found for him. After the sad loss of Rudy, they'd kept a careful eye on him for a number of months, and when a mixed breed rescue had been dropped at the practice it hadn't taken them long to know where to match her. Isla was on her best behaviour, sitting next to her owner.

Matt and Marianne were guests of honour in

the front seats. Aurora and Eli considered them family. One year on, Matt was on the road to recovery, and was back working two days a week in the practice. Their newly qualified vet, Cheryl, had shaped up better than anyone could have hoped for, and she and her family loved their move to Scotland.

The Liverpudlian half of the outside ceremony seemed to be in competition around who could wear the most spectacular hat. Aurora's mother was winning, her bright pink and navy hat obscuring some people's view of the ceremony.

Eli met the green gaze of his soon-to-be wife and mouthed one word. *Gorgeous.* Her face lit up. She glowed. He'd heard people say those words about brides before, but now he could see it with his own eyes.

As she moved alongside him he slid his arm around her waist and kissed her cheek. He just couldn't help it. They'd been through so much this year. The court case had taken its toll. Aurora had continued her counselling, and Eli had joined her when appropriate.

Even though Brandon Rivers had been convicted again, and given a much sterner sentence, there was still a sense of disquiet around them. It had led them to their latest decision to return to one of Eli's previous roles with the horses in Jerez in Spain for the next year. Hank and Bert were ready to go with them. They all needed a break—a chance for some space to let Aurora heal fully, and for their relationship to blossom into the beautiful marriage it was about to become. It was likely they would return to Scotland the following year to take over from Matt when he would finally retire.

The ceremony started and, as planned, at one point Aurora bent to pull the satin ribbon around Bert's neck that held Eli's ring, and he did the same move with Hank, to reveal her ring.

She'd never looked so bright. She'd never looked so radiant.

And as they said their vows and slipped on each other's rings Eli knew he was the luckiest man on earth.

He pulled her close to him for their kiss. 'Love you, Mrs Ferguson,' he whispered as his lips touched hers.

She wrapped her hands around his neck. 'Love you, Mr Ferguson,' she responded. Then, with a glint in her eye, she leaned back.

'I might have some news to share.'

His eyebrows raised. 'You've adopted another puppy?'

She beamed as she whispered in his ear. 'Not another puppy. But let's just say our family of four is expanding.'

Eli picked up his bride and whirled her around

as his puppies barked in excitement and the wedding guests applauded.

And it truly was a perfect day.

* * * * *

*If you enjoyed this story, check out
these other great reads from
Scarlet Wilson*

Cinderella's Kiss with the ER Doc
A Daddy for Her Twins
Nurse with a Billion Dollar Secret
Snowed In with the Surgeon

All available now!

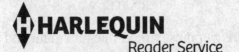

HARLEQUIN
Reader Service

Enjoyed your book?

Try the perfect subscription for Romance readers and get more great books like this delivered right to your door.

See why over 10+ million readers have tried Harlequin Reader Service.

Start with a Free Welcome Collection with free books and a gift—valued over $20.

Choose any series in print or ebook.
See website for details and order today:

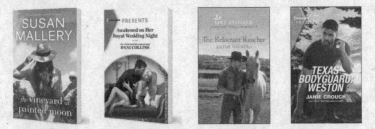

TryReaderService.com/subscriptions